Holistic Assertiveness Skills for Nurses

Empower Yourself
(and Others!)

Carolyn Chambers Clark
EdD, RN, ARNP, FAAN, HNC, DABFN, FAAIM

 Springer Publishing Company

Springer Publishing Company, Inc.
536 Broadway
New York, NY 10012-3955

Acquisitions Editor: Ruth Chasek
Production Editor: Pamela Lankas
Cover design by Joanne Honigman

03 04 05 06 07 / 5 4 3 2 1

Library of Congress Cataloging-in-Publication-Data

Clark, Carolyn Chambers.
   Holistic assertiveness skills for nurses : empower yourself and others Carolyn Chambers Clark.
      p. cm.
   Includes bibliographical references and index.
   ISBN 0-8261-1714-7
   1. Nursing—Psychological aspects—Problems, exercises, etc. 2. Holistic nursing—Problems, exercises, etc. 3. Assertiveness (Psychology)—Problems, exercises, etc.
   I. Title.

RT86.C573 2003
610.73'01'9—dc21

                                2003042787

Printed in the United States of America by Vicks Printing and Lithograph.

8

Holistic
Assertiveness Skills
for Nurses

Empower Yourself
(and Others!)

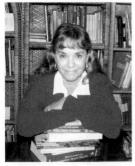

Carolyn Chambers Clark, EdD, ARNP, FAAN, HNC, DABFN, FAAIM, is on the health services doctoral faculty at Walden University and has been on the graduate and undergraduate nursing faculty at several other universities. Dr. Clark is founder of the Wellness Institute and edited *The Wellness Newsletter* for 15 years. She is founding editor of *Alternative Health Practitioner: The Journal of Complementary and Natural Care* (now called *Complementary Health Practice Review*). Her book *Wellness Practitioner: Concepts, Research and Strategies* won an *American Journal of Nursing* Book of the Year Award. She has published widely on complementary, holistic, and self-care topics for both academic and consumer audiences and is editor in chief of the *Encyclopedia of Complementary Health Practice* and author of *Integrating Complementary Health Procedures into Practice,* both *AJN* Book of the Year Award winners. Dr. Clark is certified as a holistic nurse by the American Holistic Nurses' Certification Corporation and is a Fellow and serves on the advisory board of the American Association of Integrative Medicine. She is also a diplomate of the American Board of Forensic Nursing. Dr. Clark has been a Fellow of the American Academy of Nursing since 1980 and has maintained a wellness and holistic practice with clients since 1976.

For Tony,
who empowers me

Contents

Acknowledgments

Thanks to all the nurses who have attended my assertiveness courses in the past. You've not only been an inspiration, but working with you has also enabled me to fine-tune the assertiveness materials in this book.

Introduction

Health care situations have become more complicated, more stressful. As a nurse, you probably suffer from lack of support and empowerment in the work setting. *Holistic Assertiveness Skills for Nurses* is meant to help you overcome the impulse to take out your anger and frustration about these changes on yourself and others and to help you find more assertive and empowered ways to react and be proactive. It can also help you teach clients and patients how to be more empowered and assertive in gaining access to health care.

This workbook is designed to help assess current action and change those behaviors that prevent you from feeling empowered and performing assertively. Assertive and empowerment training can assist you in learning how to express your ideas and feelings more clearly as well as tone down aggressive or attacking communications so others will be more apt to hear what you have to say.

This book focuses on the underlying causes of lack of power in the workplace and provides holistic solutions, not quick fixes that won't last. You can use all of the information in this book by yourself, in peer groups, or in formal classes to teach nurses, clients, or patients to empower themselves and become more assertive.

This book provides specific information and exercises to help stop

- turning anger inward
- feeling sabotaged and unable to fight back
- taking stress out on others
- complaining and blaming
- being hooked on helping

Once you have these basic skills, you can begin

- defining who you are and what you want
- calling upon energetic resources
- saying no to impossible demands and yes to your needs
- refusing to perpetuate patriarchy and oppression
- accepting your power to heal and be healed

This workbook has been designed to meet the needs of nurses in a variety of settings—from the individual nurse to the basic and graduate academic classroom, to peer support groups in the workplace, to continuing education workshops. It is focused on assertive skills in the work setting, not on therapy for learners who have severe anxiety, aggression, or mental health problems. If you have more complex problems, seek professional counseling or psychotherapy.

WHY A WORKBOOK FORMAT?

This book is full of exercises to help you integrate the information needed to empower yourself and others. The written exercises are crucial to attaining behavior change. Completing the exercises is important for a number of reasons. This book takes the stand that assertive behavior is learned behavior. Assertiveness is a skill, like giving an injection or taking a nursing history. Like those skills, assertiveness requires adequate and systematic practice. When you only *think* about things, there is often a tendency to forget important points or to find it difficult to focus on the topic at hand and to become bogged down in side issues. Writing your thoughts down can overcome these difficulties. Writing ideas on paper reinforces them in your mind. It also provides a permanent record for you to refer to and gives you a benchmark that will allow you to see later on how far you've come since you began your empowerment journey.

WAYS THIS BOOK CAN BE USED

You can use this book for self-study, or you may choose to gather informally with a group of peers to complete the exercises. Nursing faculty may decide to improve their own and their students' assertive skills by developing a workshop and using this book as a basis for a study and work program. The book can also be used as the text for a nursing leadership course for basic or graduate students.

ASSESSMENT IS AN IMPORTANT PART OF THE LEARNING PROCESS

Whether you use this book as an individual or in a group, assessment is an important part of the learning process. You will find it useful to assess the assertive behavior of yourself or other learners in order to zero in on the types of situations that create assertion problems. No one is assertive at all times in all situations.

Preassessment will help you to select relevant exercises as well as to individualize work on exercises by dividing larger classes into small groups, each working on a different aspect of assertion or empowerment. The directions for each exercise should be stated clearly enough in this book so that small groups can practice them without assistance.

WHY ROLE-PLAYING PRACTICE IS IMPORTANT

Practice is important. At first, making more assertive responses than you are used to making will seem foreign and strange. If you work with a colleague, saying and repeating responses, you will soon overcome this reaction and will feel more confident as the new behavior becomes part of you.

WHY IT'S IMPORTANT TO WORK WITH A PARTNER

A partner can assist you in this empowerment process by making comments such as "Try it again," "That was good," "Don't smile when you say you're angry," and so on. You will need to coach your partner about what kind of comments are helpful to you and when. The second reason it is important to work with a peer is that you will need a source of emotional support when you begin to change your behavior. At that point, you will hear others try to convince you in both subtle and direct ways to remain as you are and not become assertive or empowered. You can help your colleague feel more confident about changing behavior because you will be going through the same process and will understand the resistance others use to keep you disempowered.

STARTING A PEER SUPPORT GROUP

Whether you read this book on your own or attend a workshop or class on the topic, it is suggested that you find a small group of nurses in your work or school setting who wish to improve their assertive skills. As a group, you can provide even more support and assistance for each other. Try to meet weekly to practice role-playing situations in which you find it difficult to be assertive. Having a number of other supportive nurses available to give you feedback and coach you about how you sound or present yourself can be an effective learning experience.

Learning to be empowered and assertive is a goal that requires time, practice, and ongoing hard work. Try not to become disappointed in yourself if you are not able to be totally assertive the first or second time you try out a new behavior. You will improve if you keep working at it. To begin, choose a fairly simple, low-threat situation, one that does not have a long history of defeat. You want to build in success and thereby enhance your self-esteem. Choose a situation that includes only one other person and that can be focused on a small task or brief structured interchange to enhance your chances of success.

Although you can learn a lot by reading the material in this book and completing the exercises, in most cases you will need at least one partner to practice the skills so you can make them part of you.

If you're working with a larger peer group, divide learners into groups of three. One person practices using assertive behavior, the second serves as the target, and the third observes and evaluates the interaction using the Assertive Evaluation Criteria on page 103. Have members rotate roles, replaying the entire interchange three times or until all three are satisfied with the outcome.

WHY I WROTE THIS BOOK

I'm Carolyn Chambers Clark, a nurse practitioner with a doctorate in education, who is certified as a holistic nurse. I've also been teaching wellness, empowerment, and assertiveness skills to nurses for more than 25 years and wrote my first assertiveness text and first started offering workshops and consultation on the subject in 1977. Since then I have learned a lot that might be helpful to you. I'm going to be your coach on your journey to empowerment.

You will have your ups and downs on this journey, so when you experience additional stress, remind yourself of where you started by examining your written responses to the beginning exercises. This will provide perspective and can provide the encouragement you need to move on.

You can also contact me at cccwellness@earthlink.net for consultation. You can keep up on my latest books in related areas, scheduled workshops, or consultation availability by going to my Web site at http://home.earthlink.net/~cccwellness

Whether I hear from you or not, I wish you well on your journey to empowerment!

Carolyn Chambers Clark

Carolyn Chambers Clark, EdD, ARNP, FAAN, HNC, FAAIM

A Note for Teachers: Using This Book in the Classroom

It will be difficult for you as a faculty member or facilitator to teach assertiveness to others unless you can consistently and comfortably assert yourself with learners. Your behavior serves as a model for students. telling student nurses or graduate nurses to be assertive and then avoiding confrontations or attacking learners subtly or directly will result in negative learning experiences for all involved.

For this reason, it is wise to work through the book yourself prior to giving a course or workshop on empowerment or assertiveness. If this is not feasible, consider hiring a nurse who is skilled in assertiveness or obtain consultation. Facilitators of workshops or individual learning programs should have an advanced nursing degree or be certified by a state or national professional society in the skill. If you don't meet these qualifications, seek out supervision from the nurse who does and whose effectiveness as a facilitator has been evaluated.

If you are conducting a small workshop or course on assertiveness and leadership, you may wish to divide learners into groups of three. One person practices using assertive behavior, the second serves as the target, and the third observes and evaluates the interaction using the Assertive Evaluation Criteria. Have members rotate roles, replaying the entire interchange three times or until all three participants are satisfied with the outcome.

You can circulate among groups and provide feedback and coaching. With larger groups, you may find that modeling or demonstrating the exercise yourself by role-playing with a participant is a more efficient use of your time. You can also prepare role-play situations in advance (the book suggest quite a few practice examples) and show them during class.

As with learning any skill, it is important to actually practice the skill. Learners must actually say the words and complete the actions. If you have a class that spans a semester, assign pairs or triads to practice what was observed during class before the next session or workshop and report their findings at the beginning of the next session. When conducting a 2- or 3-day workshop, participants can be asked to read portions of the book prior to and between workshop days. This will leave the actual workshop time free for practice.

In teaching these skills, learning experiences will be most successful if learners have the freedom to choose whether to participate, and if those who seem to require psychotherapy rather than assertiveness training are so counseled. In addition, be sure you are able to recognize easily the differences and relationships between assertion, aggression, and the rights of others. In all cases, use this book responsibly and carefully.

Use the following teaching strategies for the most beneficial results:

1. Be firm with participants about practice exercises. Those who are most in need of assertiveness and empowerment skills may be the least likely to volunteer for role-playing. Check to be sure that no participant is overlooked or overprotected during role-playing segments. If you are not skilled in setting up, facilitating, and evaluating role-playing situations, obtain training or call in a consultant to co-teach the course.

2. If participants seem highly anxious about their performance in front of you on any of the exercises, get them involved in working with other learners who have role-playing and assertiveness skills. Once they have attained some comfort working with peers, remember to return to them and engage them in role-playing with you. Remind them of their assessment in the area of difficulty with authority figures and their need to work on this aspect of assertiveness.

3. Participants may become discouraged when they first practice assertiveness responses. Be sure to provide frequent and positive feedback for any approximations to assertion. To increase confidence and skill, point out at least one positive difference or behavior for each participant. Some comments to use are, "Good, see that eye contact on the videotape. You've improved," "Your voice is much firmer," or, "Your body looks more relaxed now." In addition, it is often useful to ask participants how they like their presentations, for example, "How did that feel to you" or "What would you like to change about your performance?"

4. Occasionally participants may get tears in their eyes or state, "I can't do this." Avoid focusing on the tears or the motivation

behind the resistance or playing into the helplessness aspect of participant behavior. One way to handle is to ask another participant to help the anxious person, for example, by saying, "Ginny, you're good at saying this; go over by Rita and coach her." Another way might be to say, "You can do it; we just saw you being firm about that with Hilda," or "You're doing fine; give it a try; I'll help you." Give the direct and nonverbal message: "You can learn this. It may be difficult, but I [we] will help you by helping you to practice."

5. After praising a participant for a performance on tape or in a live role-play situation, choose no more than two simple modes of behavior and ask that person to concentrate on them for the next role-play or for the replay of that situation. For example, "Your tone of voice is much firmer. Next time, concentrate on looking her right in the eye when you speak to her."

6. Be very specific when providing feedback to a participant who is role-playing. Many participants benefit from being told exactly what to say to their role partner, especially when they get into difficulty and look to you for assistance. For example, you might say, "Tell her you can't work overtime and keep telling her until she stops asking," or "Look her right in the eye and tell her you're expecting her to be on time for work."

7. Dispute comments from participants that convey attitudes and misconceptions that inhibit them from asserting themselves. For example, if a participant says, "I don't really mind staying late and working overtime," say, "You have a right to leave work on time if you choose to."

8. Keep checking to ensure that participants understand and use terms appropriately. They need to use the terms assertive, aggressive, and acquiescent/avoiding in the same way with one another and with you. If you hear anyone misusing terms, step in and clarify the definitions.

1

Are You Divesting Yourself of Power?

Self-development is a higher duty than self-sacrifice.
—Elizabeth Cady Stanton

There are numerous situations that can divest you of power . . . if you let them.

How do you know if you're living a quality life, one that empowers you? Here are a few questions to ask yourself and help you evaluate that (the more yes answers, the less your life is empowering):

- I have trouble putting my own needs before others; this leads to feeling frustrated and resentful about my commitments.
- I feel drained by a long list of "things to do" that I never seem to finish.
- I'd like to spend more time taking care of my spiritual side (meditation, prayer, finding a life purpose), but life keeps getting in the way.
- I feel isolated or disconnected from others and wish I had a deeper connection with a community of like-minded people.
- I feel trapped by money and can't leave a job I hate because of finances.
- I'd like to slow down, but peace seems an unattainable goal.

If you had even one yes, you are divesting yourself of power and may want to think about what to do to empower yourself. Major divestitures of power include job stress, anger, sabotage, complaining, blaming, and overhelping. This chapter includes ways to assess how these variables may be disabling you and preventing you from feeling empowered.

JOB STRESS AND BURNOUT

Job stress can lead to burnout and divestiture of empowerment. *Burnout* is a prolonged response to chronic emotional and interpersonal stressors and is defined by the dimensions of exhaustion, cynicism, and inefficacy (Maslach, Schaufeli, & Leiter, 2001). Burnout has also been defined as the state of being worn out by excessive or improper use, fatigue, numbness, depression and paralysis (Broffman, 2001). Occupational stressors can lead t burnout (Payne, 2001; Davis & Thornburn, 1999; Lewis, 1999; Linn, Sandifer & Stein, 1985; Lindberg, 1999; MacDonald et al., 2001; McDonough, 2000; Parry-Jones et al., 1988).

The costs of job stress in lost productivity and health care are estimated to be $300 billion annually (Rosch, 2002). As well, adverse work and environmental conditions also predict hypertension (Fauvel et al., 2001), occupational injuries (Melamed, Yekultieli, Froom, Kristal-Bonch, & Ribak, 1999) and motor vehicle accidents (Norris, Matthews, & Riad, 2000), so making the work site less distressing can save employers many dollars.

Stress and Burnout in Physicians

It would be logical to expect that physician burnout would be related to heavy on-call responsibility, overload, poor job control, social circumstances outside the workplace, and health behaviors. That may not be the case. A large study of physicians found that teamwork had the greatest effect on sickness absence in physicians but not in controls. Working in poorly functioning teams was more stressful and led to more sick leave than any other factor (Broffman, 2001; Kivimaki et al., 2001).

Broffman (2001) discussed characteristics of physicians, especially physician executives, that make them prime candidates for burnout. Perfectionism is one quality that exacts a toll on individual physicians and can contribute to burnout. When physician executives function at a level that is less than perfect they are especially hard on themselves. This can lead to feelings of depression, self-doubt, and low self-esteem. They work harder to prevent failure, become fatigued, and perform even more poorly. They end up venting their frustration on their colleagues, support staff, and families. This can lead to isolation, a direct route to burnout. Doubt and guilt due to an exaggerated sense of responsibility can lead to a workaholic syndrome with restriction of leisure and family time, the very activities that could calm and soothe.

Burnout in Nurses

Many forces can bring about burnout in nurses. Health care settings and third-party payors influence the length of hospital stay, making it difficult for nurses to evaluate whether they've made an impact on patient or client health-care outcomes. Government eligibility criteria may force nurses to deny care to uninsured or low-income families which can lead to bitterness and cynicism in nurses. The institutional system contributes to burnout by providing insufficient staff or insufficient or faulty equipment, by mandating overtime, and by asking nurses to lower their standards to accommodate the employer's financial agendas. Mixed messages abound: Give quality care but exercise cost containment on supplies. Give quality care but do it for an unmanageable number of acutely ill patients.

Many nursing tasks are stressful, too (Parry-Jones et al., 1998). Nurses are expected to deal with situations most of the public would find uncomfortable and frightening, such as, handling contaminated body fluids, being assaulted by an angry or confused patient, caring for babies born to drug-addicted mothers (Cullen, 1995) and lifting heavy patients (Linton, 2001; MacDonald et al., 2001). Nurses in intensive care units can experience post-traumatic stress disorder after being confronted with seriously injured, mutilated, and dying patients, corpses, and their own anxiety and helplessness (Teegen & Muller, 2000).

Working with unlicensed assistive personnel can lead to job dissatisfaction. When nurses believe these workers are "undependable" or "do not have the knowledge to interpret a situation" nurse job dissatisfaction increases (Fletcher, 2001).

Burnout in nursing is of individual *and* organizational concern because it affects well-being, job performance, absenteeism, and turnover (Kilfedder, Power, & Wells, 2001). A study of community mental-health nurses exemplifies burnout issues similar to nurses in many settings. As a result of increasing workload and increasing administrative demands and lack of resources, stress and burnout increased. Specific stressors included time management, inappropriate referrals, safety issues, role conflict, role ambiguity, lack of supervision, not having enough time for personal study, general working conditions, and lack of funding (Edwards, Burnard, Coyle, Fothergill, & Hannigan, 2000). Lack of communication and career development can also lead to burnout (Rout, 2000).

JOB STRESS CAN LEAD TO PHYSICAL SYMPTOMS

Studies have found that job stress is associated with coronary disease risk and psychosomatic distress (Steffy & Jones, 1988), with disorders in blood coagulation and fibrinolysis (von Kanel et al., 2001), and with higher blood pressure (Fauvel et al, 2001). Job dissatisfaction, monotonous tasks, poor work relationships, high job demands and high stress were correlated with risk for back pain (Linton, 2001; MacDonald et al., 2001) and neck and shoulder pain (Palmer et al., 2001; Lundberg, 1999).

Job stress in nurses is related to headaches, upset stomach, insomnia, gas and bloated feelings, changes in bowel movement, early morning sickness, loss of appetite, dizziness during the day, nervousness or shakiness inside, and inability to relax (Jamal & Baba, 2000); sleeping problems, tension headache, chronic fatigue and palpitations, regular alcohol drinking, heavy smoking, and frequent use of tranquilizers and sleeping pills (Piko, 1999). Another study found that full-time nurses were 1 1/2 times more likely to be a recent nonmedical drug user if they had a high strain job (Storr, Trinkoff, & Anthony, 1999). Trauma exposure and subsequent post-traumatic stress disorder result in significantly more depressive symptoms and deficiencies in emotional competence in nurses who work in ICUs (Teegen & Muller, 2000).

Having little control over a job has been linked with upper respiratory illnesses and lowered immune function (Schaubroeck, Jones, & Xie, 2001). Job stress may be the mediating factor between smoking and the development of peptic ulcers (Shigemi, Mino, & Tsuda, 1999).

The first step in the process of finding out what situations divest you of power is to examine the ways you deal with anger and how each affects you. Some of the specific ways you may be divesting yourself of power include turning anger inward, feeling sabotaged and unable to fight back, taking stress out on others, complaining and blaming, and being hooked on helping. Let's take a look at each of these behaviors.

TURNING ANGER INWARD IS COSTLY

Everyone gets angry. It's a human response to frustration and stress and there's no sense denying it exists, even if some people who are important in your life pretend it doesn't. Often, hurt and suffering are under the anger. The anger is just a cover for these more basic feelings. It may be stress that is building, not anger, but it is the anger that is expressed.

If you're okay with getting angry, you can express it, release it, or let it go. If anger is not acceptable to you, it's likely you'll turn it against yourself. A common result of turning anger against yourself can be the development of back problems (Linton, 2001).

Hay (2000) takes a more metaphysical look at back problems. This theory states that the good and bad in life and "dis-ease" result from thought patterns. The negative thought patterns are the ones that result in dis-ease. An occasional negative thought isn't going to hurt. It is the consistent negative thought patterns that create a negative body pattern.

In this framework, anger at lack of financial support may result in lower back pain. Wanting someone to "get off my back," may result in middle back pain. Feeling angry about being unloved may result in upper back pain.

It is not only back pain that results from turning anger inward. In Hay's framework, headaches may be due to invalidating the self, self-criticism, and fear. Neck pain may result from inflexibility, not wanting to see "what's back there." Shoulder pain may mean an inability to carry experiences joyously, which makes life a burden. Stomach problems may be viewed as a result of dread, fear of the new, and inability to assimilate new ideas. If you can't sleep, it could be because you don't trust your life process. Gas and bloating may be undigested ideas. Constipation may occur because you're stuck in the past, unable to release old ideas or memories, and diarrhea may be due to fear and rejection. Self-hatred and extreme fear may lead to lack of appetite. Dizziness may be the result of scattered thinking and a refusal to look at what's happening to you. Nervousness may be due to rushing and struggling, not trusting. Fatigue may be the result of boredom, resistance, and lack of love for your work. Depression may be anger you don't feel comfortable expressing and could be due to hopelessness. Respiratory illness may be due to grief and to fear of taking in life. Ulcers may be due to a strong belief of not being good enough so that in effect, you "eat away" at yourself.

If you do turn anger inward, it's probably because you're afraid of your own anger and don't want to have a confrontation with another person. This is something you no doubt learned in your family and had reinforced in school and work situations.

If you're a woman, you probably learned that expressing your anger is inappropriate (Brown & Gilligan, 1992). Even if you overcame that myth, when you tried to express your anger you may have been called a bitch, a shrew, a man-hater, unfeminine, or other unflattering names.

If you're a man, you may have more experience expressing your anger, but you may also have learned to be physically aggressive. Acting out your aggression has a negative side and can lead to feeling guilty.

Either situation can result in turning your anger on yourself and so can perfectionism. Most of us have learned very early to please our parents, to be "nice," conform to other peoples' expectations, and try to be perfect. School measures that perfection by giving us grades. "I got an A, that means I'm better than you are." This compulsion for rating ourselves as better or worse can stay forever. It's a very destructive idea.

No matter what your work setting, situations that anger you are a major source of stress and can divest you of power. Anger has enormous costs. It can hurt you physically if you turn it inward, and it can damage your relationships if you spew it out. Take a look at Exercise 1 and identify the situations that anger you.

EXERCISE 1 Anger Triggers

Directions: Below you'll find some situations that can trigger anger and divest you of power. Place a check in front of the events that anger you.

___ people not carrying their load
___ belligerence or disrespect from others
___ the stronger taking advantage of the weaker
___ power-hungry people
___ unfaithfulness
___ family members who don't help out around the house
___ half-finished jobs that I must redo
___ family members or people at work who leave inappropriate messages
___ feeling sick or tired
___ being overworked
___ fear of physical violence
___ bad work assignments
___ situations that slow me down from reaching my goal
___ inadequate job training
___ people who say one thing and do another
___ insufficient time for discussion

(continued)

EXERCISE 1 (*continued*)

___ being asked to do something I don't want to do and doing it anyway
___ not being offered a choice or having input when the outcome affects me
___ when a situation is overwhelming and I'm not able to control it
___ not being listened to
___ when I'm afraid
___ other: fill in the blank _____

_____
_____

Now that you've identified situations that anger you, take a look at them and see how many variables you are reacting to. Were you surprised at how many situations angered you? If you checked more than one or two items, you could be carrying around a lot of unresolved anger. Over time, that could hurt your physical body, your mental attitude, and your soul. If you keep reading along and doing the exercises, you will learn more about your anger.

Identifying your anger and its effects is the first step toward changing. Have confidence.

If you suffer from job stress and have no healthy outlet for your anger, you may find yourself suffering from headaches, stomachaches, other aches and pains, fatigue, palpitations, depression, or hopelessness. You may gain weight from stuffing in food to hold your anger in. You may also use drugs, alcohol, or heavy smoking. Although these measures may help for a while, they won't work for long because they're only focused on the symptom, not on the underlying cause. That is why a holistic approach is needed.

Sandra Thomas' groundbreaking research on women and anger (1993) found that neither turning anger in nor turning it outward in aggressive outbursts was helpful. Both responses can catch you in an endless cycle of low self-esteem and depression that can worsen anger because you never deal with the issues that evoke it.

Take a few minutes to complete the exercise below to help you identify anger you may be turning inward.

EXERCISE 2 Turning Anger Inward

Directions: Check off all the signs that indicate you may be turning anger inward when you're stressed.

___getting down on myself or feeling demoralized
___muscular or bone aches or pains
___occupational injuries or "accidents"
___nonmedical drug use
___tension headache
___sleeping problems
___chronic fatigue
___palpitations
___drinking alcohol
___smoking
___using tranquilizers or sleeping pills
___depression
___hopelessness
___overeating
___other: (describe) _____

How many ways are you turning your anger inward? Did some of your answers surprise you? One of the major reasons you may turn your anger inward is because you feel sabotaged and unable to fight back.

FEELING SABOTAGED AND UNABLE TO FIGHT BACK

We've all felt sabotaged at times. Some of us fight back or overlook the sabotage. Others feel it like a knife in the back or in the heart, stumble and fall. Many will get up and start again. Some will not. This book is meant to help you see that everyone has this experience and to help you get up and start again.

It may happen that you feel betrayed by a colleague you trusted and confided in. Maybe your feelings of sabotage come because you thought you could count on a supervisor or boss, then found out you couldn't. It could even be a friend or family member who leads you on, then breaks your heart.

But, your heart isn't broken. It's just wounded. You can fix it.

Betrayal

A most hurtful kind of sabotage is betrayal. Exercise 3 will help you get in touch with, and begin to understand, situations that have sabotaged you through betrayal.

EXERCISE 3 Feeling Betrayed

Directions:

1. Find a quiet place and write about one time when you felt betrayed by someone.
2. Write for at least 15 minutes, paying no attention to the words. Just write.
3. Avoid censoring what you write. Pour your feelings onto the page.
4. Once you've written all you can, go back and read it.
5. Add anything you want to add now, but don't change what you wrote before.
6. Put it away for a week, then look at it and see what you can learn from what you've written.
7. Some questions to ask yourself are:
   a. Why did that situation bother me so much?
   b. What was really going on between us?
   c. How is what happened like what used to happen in my family?
   d. What is underneath my anger? Is it fear, insecurity, regret, guilt, or some other feeling?
   e. What would have to happen so I could experience those feelings under the anger?
   f. What can I do make that happen?

Maybe no one else is sabotaging you. It could be that you sabotage your own success.

Self-Esteem and Self-Sabotage

Why would you want to sabotage yourself? Low self-esteem is one answer. Self-esteem is your self-confidence, self-worth, and self-respect. If you have low self-esteem you have difficulty accepting compliments and having confidence in what you say or do. You probably avoid eye contact, turn red easily, and get a "shame attack." If you have low self-esteem, it is probably because you weren't valued by your caregivers. They did not esteem you in an appropriate way. In neglecting to value you, they abused you, even if they didn't mean to.

If you were abused or neglected in your family of origin, you probably abuse or neglect yourself. The key to elevating your self-esteem is the willingness to take responsibility for your thoughts, feelings, and actions.

Self-esteem fluctuates depending on your life experiences. It is an ongoing evaluation of yourself and your abilities. If you have low self-esteem now, take heart. You can learn to build your self-esteem, but it won't happen overnight. It will take time.

When you make the decision to value yourself, it will be easier for you to value others. As your self-esteem rises, so will your esteem of others. This change can make your relationships wonderful.

On the surface you may think you want to succeed, but underneath, old messages you learned in your family continue to operate. I call these faulty tapes. Perhaps you were told you were stupid, lazy, would never succeed, or were given some other negative message. These messages are like tapes that play in your head. They're faulty because they have nothing to do with you and everything to do with the originator of the message. They may even seem automatic, as if they turn themselves on and play and play and there is nothing you can do about it.

Take heart. There *is* something you can do about it, but first you must identify the messages and realize they are not you. They belong to someone else. Until you identify these messages, face them, and realize you are perfect and whole, you will continue to sabotage yourself.

Complete Exercise 4 to help you identify these messages.

EXERCISE 4 Identifying Your Faulty Tapes

Directions:

1. Find a quiet, safe spot where you can be alone and undisturbed. If necessary, put a note on your door—DO NOT DISTURB—or ask your house mate(s) to please respect that you need some time alone. You may wish to record the rest of these directions on a tape and play them back. That way, you can concentrate on the experience. If you do record the directions, make sure to read them slowly and in a monotone voice, pausing for several seconds at each elipsis (. . .).

2. Get a pad and a pen or pencil and take it with you . . .

3. Sit or lie down in a comfortable spot . . .

4. Kick off your shoes . . . loosen tight clothing . . . and do whatever you have to do to feel comfortable and safe . . .

5. Pay attention to your breathing . . . Give yourself a gentle suggestion to let your breath begin to move lower in your body, moving toward your center . . .

6. Picture yourself very young . . . you are back in your family . . . with your parent(s) . . .

7. What is it like to be that small child? . . . See yourself in that room . . . hear your parent(s) speaking to you or about you . . . what are the words telling you about yourself? . . .

8. Pay particular attention to the messages that are sarcastic, humiliating, hurtful, or frightening . . .

9. When you have the words well in mind, write down the messages you heard . . . write them all down so you can look at them . . . (pause for 2–5 minutes)

10. Look at your list of the messages you received from your parent(s) . . . Put a check in front of the ones that are behaviors and attitudes you want to keep in your life . . .

Save your list. Now go back and repeat this exercise, only this time, write about school experiences that led to your feeling disempowered. When you've finished, go back and write about work experiences that led to your feeling disempowered. Save these answers, too. You will be using them in later chapters.

Not being prepared, well-rested, and well-nourished or leaning too heavily on others can lead to feeling sabotaged when things don't work out the way you planned. Using crutches, such as drugs, alcohol, or heavy smoking, to get you through can end up sabotaging you because they cloud your senses or cripple your body's ability to be in tip-top form.

Once you have lost your sense of power in the situation, you are bound to feel less able to fight back. Perhaps worse, in terms of your career, it can lead to fighting back too strongly and being labeled a maverick, trouble-maker, or difficult person. Go to Exercise 5 now and find out ways you may be sabotaging yourself.

EXERCISE 5 How You Sabotage Yourself

Directions: Check off the following ways in which you sabotage yourself.

___ I hold on to old messages that tell me I'm stupid, lazy, will never be successful, or that make me feel less than whole.

___ I'm never prepared and that can make me look bad.

___ I don't get enough sleep so I feel tired and out of sorts all day.

___ I don't eat right so I can't think straight, feel weak, and don't function very well.

___ I lean on others too much and then feel heartbroken when they're not perfect.

___ I cloud my ability to think clearly by taking drugs, drinking alcohol, or heavy smoking.

Go back and look at the actions you're taking to sabotage yourself. Vow to stop doing at least one of these behaviors and find a way to keep your vow.

A first step in changing from sabotage to success is examining the relationships in your personal and work life that lead to your feeling sabotaged. It is time to ask yourself what relationships in your life make you feel sabotaged and unable to fight back. Once you have identified the relationships, try to see what it is about those situations that divest you of power.

Let's take a look at how you evaluate your personal and work life and how it could be affecting your self-esteem by looking at Exercise 6.

EXERCISE 6 How Does Your Life Affect Your Self-Esteem?

Directions: Rate your self-esteem from 1 (low self-esteem) to 5 (high self-esteem).

___ I feel satisfied with my achievements.
___ I can handle whatever situation comes along.
___ I can take and give compliments
___ I like to tell others about my accomplishments.
___ I make decisions easily based on the facts.
___ I am comfortable in new situations.
___ I look for the good in myself and others.
___ I take care of myself.
___ I take responsibility for my own actions.
___ I can ask for help without feeling guilty.
___ I think of obstacles as challenges.
___ I can see the humor in difficult situations.
___ I can express my feelings in a calm manner.
___ I like who I am and what I do.

The more 3–5 ratings you have, the higher your self-esteem. The more 1s and 2s, the lower your self-esteem.

TAKING STRESS OUT ON OTHERS

If you have low self-esteem, high stress, and few assertive skills, you may find yourself taking your feelings out on others. This is the opposite of taking your anger out on yourself by getting depressed, being down on yourself, getting sick, or using drugs or alcohol. When you take your stress out on others, you become aggressive. One kind of aggressiveness involves being directly hostile and going on the attack. Aggressive messages usually contain the word "you." It can be implied, such as "Don't shout at me!" or direct, as in "You don't know what you're talking about."

Aggressive and avoiding behaviors are related in the sense that both are the opposite of assertive behavior. If you tend to avoid situations, eventually you will have your fill and probably blow up and get angry. You may experience a buildup of angry and resentful feelings that may then erupt in emotional upset or outbursts. You may even be passive-aggressive and use subtle put-downs, nagging, calling in sick, be chronically forgetful, break confidentiality, procrastinate, fantasize and daydream, or change the subject when a confrontation is about to occur. Trying to make other people feel guilty is another example of passive-aggressive behavior. So are teasing, unfair criticism, saying yes and agreeing to a task then never acting, and appearing so fragile the other person is intimidated. Over-agreeableness or agreeing to anything so you don't rock the boat is also passive-aggressive. Complete Exercise 7 now to help you identify your aggressive behaviors.

EXERCISE 7 Identifying Your Aggressive Behaviors

Directions: Write a paragraph about the following situations. Identify how you acted aggressively either directly or indirectly. Be sure to include who was involved besides you, what you said and did, what the other person(s) said or did, and how you felt about the outcome.

Situations:

1. A time you lost your temper and blew up:

2. A time you conveniently "forgot" to do something you had promised to do:

3. A time you broke confidentiality by sharing something without checking first to make sure it was okay to share the information:

4. A time you procrastinated and prevented others from accomplishing their goals:

(continued)

EXERCISE 7 (*continued*)

5. A time you nagged someone:

6. A time you called in sick before a tense meeting or confrontation:

7. A time you either fantasized, daydreamed, or changed the subject when a confrontation was about to occur:

8. A time when you tried to make someone else feel guilty:

9. A time you criticized someone unfairly:

10. A time you teased someone:

(*continued*)

11. A time you said yes or agreed to do something, then never did it:

12. A time you spoke softly or appeared so fragile the other person was intimidated and let you have your way:

13. A time you agreed to do anything so you wouldn't rock the boat:

If you couldn't come up with an incident for at least five of the situations, you're probably not being honest or maybe you're just not in touch with your aggressiveness. Ask a colleague, friend, or family member for ideas or feedback. Once you've identified the situations, write a paragraph about each occasion.

COMPLAINING AND BLAMING

There is nothing wrong with complaining. It can be an effective tool if used appropriately. Complaining is not empowering when it becomes an act unto itself. Complaints can only empower you if they are a springboard to positive action.

Scenario:

Sarah had come to hate her job. She could barely drag herself out of bed on Monday morning and called in sick as often as she could. On days when she had to go to work, she moped and procrastinated, barely accomplishing her assigned tasks, putting her job in jeopardy. She was curt and snide with her colleagues, and let them do most of the work. Whenever she had a chance, she complained about her job, her boss, her colleagues and just about everything else. When she went home at night, she was so tired she could barely eat dinner. Her stomach was upset and she had headaches almost every night. She'd started drinking a bottle of wine at night and taking sleeping pills to get to sleep. She's had five colds this winter and can't seem to shake the last one and she coughs and feels feverish most of the time. She has diarrhea one day and constipation the next and she feels dizzy sometimes.

It is pretty clear that Sarah is in burnout. She is no longer functioning at her level of competence and her focus is almost entirely on complaining. She has taken her anger and converted it to complaining so she has no energy for anything else. Complete Exercise 8 to assess your complaining behaviors.

EXERCISE 8 Complaining

Directions: Describe one time when all you did was complain. Write about that time and what was happening. Tell what happened and who was there. Write about exactly what was said and what the outcome was. When you're finished writing, set it aside. You may want to come back to this situation in a later chapter.

Write about a situation when you complained:

Blaming can also be disempowering. Not much good can be said about blaming, yet most of us look around for someone to blame when something goes wrong: "It's your fault!" "No, it's his fault!" "No, hers!" When it comes down to it, what does it matter whose fault it is? Even if we could determine scientifically whose fault something is, what good can that do us?

Blaming can do a lot of harm. First of all, the ones who are blamed are left feeling guilty and maybe even paranoid that everyone has ganged up on them. This can do damage to group cohesiveness and the ability to work effectively together.

When you're in pain, you may want to find someone to blame. "Who did this to me?" is a common question. The impulse to blame someone else lies at the heart of chronic anger. When you can identify a source to blame, it is all too easy to start discharging your anger at that source. If someone did something to you, the next step is to identify yourself as a victim. You are under siege and threatened, alone and undefended.

There can be a sense of relief in blaming. When you can find someone else to be responsible for what happens to you, it takes the focus away from your pain and puts it on your suffering. This blocks you from experiencing stress and for a brief time you may even feel better.

But the relief is short-lived and it's an invalid strategy. No one else can be responsible for your pain. It's your pain and you are responsible for how you feel. You determine whether your needs are met, whether you're in pain, whether your relationships work out, and what you do with your life. All this is determined by the choices you make. Complete Exercise 9 now and examine your blaming behaviors.

EXERCISE 9 Blaming

Directions: Write a paragraph about each of the statements that follow, giving at least one example for each item of when you did blame someone else.

1. I am the only one who really knows what I need so there's no sense blaming others.

2. It isn't anybody's responsibility to take care of me.

3. As long as there is someone else with me, there's bound to be conflict.

4. If I'm unhappy, it means I have to find a better way to get what I want and avoid pain.

BEING HOOKED ON HELPING

Helping can be positive, but being hooked on helping can be detrimental. You're hooked on helping when you become overinvolved in "taking care of" others. Did you ever stop to think that all the energy you're putting in to help others and doing for them is depriving you of your own power? Are you hooked on helping? What if all that energy went into teaching others to be assertive and self-responsible?

Scenario:

Skilled, experienced nurses work for a large city hospital. They make a good salary, but the working conditions are poor. The administration is disorganized and nonsupportive (even after many meetings to discuss staff dissatisfaction), the units are understaffed, supplies are low, and the nursing staff suffers from low morale. A union organizer is trying to unite nurses to take a stand and, if necessary, to strike for better conditions.

Passive response:
Adrian is trapped by her helping motives. She tells her peers it would be selfish to talk about taking any action that could lead to a strike and leave the patients in the lurch. Adrian tells her colleagues that they must put up with poor working conditions and low morale for the sake of the patients. Confrontation frightens her, and she is convinced that nurses have to think of others first and keep peace.

Passive-aggressive response:
Beverly feels helpless and sorry for her patients and herself. She reacts by blaming her colleagues, neglecting the patients she has been assigned, and developing a "things will never change" attitude.

Aggressive response:
Wanda is unable to directly face her anger. Instead, she gets labeled an "angry bitch" by the administration and some of her colleagues. She overreacts and makes hostile threats, going right to the top administrator and screaming at him. The end result is that administration is now even less likely to deal with nursing issues.

Assertive response:
Susan believes in an active response, too. She is concerned with patient welfare (short-term goal), but is able to see the larger picture that taking the risk and possibly striking could better conditions at the hospital (long-term goal). She calls a meeting and expresses her concern to her colleagues, urging them to strike. "We must stand united," she tells them, "if we want to make a real impact and get conditions to improve." When some of the nurses express worry about patient welfare and fear of retaliation, she keeps the topic on course and continues to urge her colleagues to organize by taking a strong, but fair stand. She asks her peers, "Are we really helping people by taking care of the things that cause them discomfort? What

price do we pay when we feel burned out, obligated, and resentful?

Are you hooked on helping? A lot of health care workers, mothers, women, and even a lot of men are. If you're hooked on helping, you get upset if your supervisees, clients, or family members don't take responsibility for their behavior, but you often end up doing the work yourself, then complaining that "no one around here does anything right!" You may find it hard to set limits on intrusions and demands and think you have to help anyone who asks for help.

Take a look at the Hooked on Helping situations that follow and judge the extent to which you are stuck helping instead of teaching others to be more assertive and holistically promoting their own health. Choose the response that comes closest to how you believe you would act in each situation, then check the key to see how hooked on helping you are.

Situation 1:

You've been hoping to finish a required work report that is immensely important to you. Some friends drop by unexpectedly, but you need to finish the report. Do you
A. Invite your colleagues to stay
B. Ignore your colleague and work on the report after giving them coffee
C. Explain you're in the middle of an important report and arrange to see them at a mutually convenient time.
D. Snap at them for not having called first.

Situation 2:

You are enjoying a convention in New Orleans and are staying with a colleague. You want to sample the local fine food, but your colleague insists you visit her parents. Do you
A. Decide to have dinner with your colleague's parents so you don't hurt their feelings
B. Make fun of the meal and stamp off to bed early
C. Go to bed without dinner, claiming to be ill, then sneak out for a meal
D. Tell your colleague you appreciate her helpfulness, but that one of the reasons you came to New Orleans was to enjoy the cuisine, then suggest all of you got out to eat instead.

Situation 3:

Your 11-year-old client usually takes the bus to your session, but today she wants you to give her a ride and refuses to come to the session unless you drive her. Do you
A. Threaten to call her parents and have them drive her
B. Say you won't drive her, then change you mind after she sulks and threatens you
C. Tell her to take the bus as usual
D. Have pangs of guilt about being neglectful and then drive her to school.

Situation 4:

You've agreed to fill in for a colleague, but you get news that a course you're taking is having an exam tomorrow and you need to study. Do you
A. Feel a headache coming on and call in sick at your place of work
B. Realize that the least you can do is cover for your colleague even though your schoolwork will suffer
C. Tell your colleague it's not fair of her to force you to fill in now that you have a test
D. Tell your colleague exactly what happened, that you'll call two friends and see if they can fill in, and then feel good because you've been honest and fair.

Situation 5:

Your boss asks you to work late again even though you don't get paid overtime and it's the one night you have tickets for the ballet. Do you
A. Agree to work, then yell at an assistant and daydream through the late time
B. Tell your boss he has some nerve
C. Feign illness, then go to the ballet
D. Tell the boss that you'd be glad to help out another time, but that you have tickets for the ballet that night.

Key to Rating Your Responses

Situation 1:   C = 5 points; all others = 0 points

A.You'll probably feel resentful later on and that's not healthy for you or your relationships.
B. Passive-aggressive. You're taking hostility out inappropriately. Be honest.
C. Assertive. Hurrah for you!
D. You may lose them as friends.

Situation 2:   D = 5 points; all others = 0 points

A. Hooked on helping.
B. Aggressive. Is a tantrum next?
C. You may feel guilty later, especially if you're caught, then what will you say?
D. Assertive!

Situation 3:   C = 5 points; all others = 0 points

A. Aggressive. You're going too far and may push her to further manipulations.
B. Avoiding. You'll probably be resentful later. You're hooked on helping.
C. Assertive. Congratulations!
D. You aren't being neglectful, but you're hooked on helping.

Situation 4:   D = 5 points; all others = 0 points

A. You may feel guilty later or lose self-respect.
B. Hooked on helping.
C. Aggressive. You may get retaliated against.
D. Assertive. Good for you!

Situation 5:   D = 5 points; all others = 0 points

A. Passive-aggressive response. You're not really working and you're taking out your anger on someone else instead of directing it toward your goal.
B. Aggressive and may get you fired.

C. Avoiding. You have just lied to your boss. There may be guilt involved in this one.
D. Assertive. You've given a very good reason for not working and haven't backed down to manipulation.

Add up your total points.
15 = you couldn't ask for more. You are on your way to assertiveness, but watch out for other situations. No one is 100% assertive in all situations.
10–15 = you're not completely hooked on helping, but be sure to do all the exercises in this book and find a supportive peer group to work with.
Less than 10 = consider the price you pay when you do things at the expense of your own happiness. Complete all the exercises in this book, join a supportive peer group, and take an assertiveness workshop or two until you can act assertively and feel good about it.

If you're not hooked on helping, you learned to separate your responsibility for what you did from taking responsibility for what others did. You also learned to value your time and experience and to set limits on the intrusions of others. If you're in the helping professions or are a manager, you also learned to provide your clients, patients, or supervisees with guidance and expertise to help them make informed decisions, and even to follow through, asking them how their self-care or career growth programs are going. One thing you did not do was take responsibility for whether they followed through. You learned that each person can only be responsible for one person: himself or herself.

If you're hooked on helping, it is probably because you learned this behavior early in life. This is common if you came from a family where you were abused or your parents were addicted to alcohol or drugs. It's also common in a family where one member needed a lot of care and you were designated (by yourself or someone else) to take care of that person, even though it is inappropriate for a child to be totally responsible for what happens to a sibling or parent. Guilt may have factored in, too, when you started to believe that you were responsible for someone else's behavior, even though that's impossible and inappropriate. It may even surprise you to think or hear that the people in your care can take responsibility for their own lives and should be encouraged to do so. It's amazing how much progress others can make once they are clearly told that both the choices and the consequences of their choices are theirs, not yours.

Whatever your situation, if you are overhelping, *boundaries* were and are not clearly defined. You learned early to get so involved with others and their needs that you may have lost your identity and stopped taking care of yourself in order to help others. Go to Exercise 10 to see if you're hooked on helping.

EXERCISE 10 My Boundaries

Directions: Rate yourself from 1 (never) to 10 (always) on each statement below by circling your level of competence for each item

	Never	Seldom		Sometimes		Often		Always	
1. I can separate other people's feelings and thoughts from my own.	1	2	3	4	5	6	7	8	9	10
2. I believe I am responsible for my own thoughts, feelings, and actions.	1	2	3	4	5	6	7	8	9	10
3. I believe other people are responsible for what they think, feel, and do with their lives.	1	2	3	4	5	6	7	8	9	10
4. I am autonomous and independent.	1	2	3	4	5	6	7	8	9	10
5. I can communicate my rationale for what I value and believe.	1	2	3	4	5	6	7	8	9	10
6. I can negotiate with others to make sure their needs and mine are satisfied.	1	2	3	4	5	6	7	8	9	10
7. I allow others to have their own values and beliefs.	1	2	3	4	5	6	7	8	9	10
8. I ask for help when I need it.	1	2	3	4	5	6	7	8	9	10
9. I ask others when they need help and respect their answer.	1	2	3	4	5	6	7	8	9	10
10. I believe all people are of equal value.	1	2	3	4	5	6	7	8	9	10

Analysis: The more answers you rated 1 through 7, the lower your self-esteem. The more answers rated 8 through 10, the higher your self-esteem. If you have low self-esteem, you will have difficulty taking good care of yourself.

You have now completed the introduction and assessment portions of this book. If you read the information above and completed all the exercises, you now have some basic skills to help evaluate situations in which you may be disempowering yourself. Now it's time to go on and learn specific empowering skills.

REFERENCES

Brown L., Gilligan, C. (1992). *Meeting at the crossroads: Women's psychology and girls' development.* Cambridge, MA: Harvard University Press.

Cullen A. (1995). Burnout: Why do we blame the nurse? *American Journal of Nursing, 95,* 23–28.

Davis B., & Thorburn, B. (1999). Quality of nurses' work life: Strategies for enhancement. *Canadian Journal of Nurse Leadership, 12*(4), 11–15.

Edwards, D., Burnard, P., Coyle, D., Fothergill, A. & Hannigan, B. (2000). Stress and burnout in community mental health nursing: a review of the literature. *Journal of Psychiatric and Mental Health Nursing, 7*(1), 7–14.

Fauvel, J. P., Quelin, P., Ducher, M., Rakotomalala, H., Laville, M. (2001). Perceived job stress but not individual cardiovascular reactivity to stress is related to higher blood pressure at work. *Hypertension, 38*(1),71–75.

Ginexi, E. M., Howe, G. W., Caplan, R. D. (2000). Depression and control beliefs in relation to reemployment: what are the directions of effect? *Journal of Occupational Health Psychology, 5*(3), 323–336.

Hay, L. (2000). *Heal your body: The mental causes for physical illness and the metaphysical way to overcome them.* Carlsbad, CA: Hay House.

Jamal, M., & Baba, V. V. (2000). Job stress and burnout among Canadian managers and nurses: an empirical examination. *Canadian Journal of Public Health, 91,* 454–458.

Kilfedder, C. J., Power, K. G., & Wells, T. J. (2001). Burnout in psychiatric nursing. *Journal of Advanced Nursing, 34,* 383–396.

Kivimaki, M., Sutinen, R., Elovainio, M., Vahtera, J., Rasanen, K., Toyry, S., Ferrie, J. E., & Firth-Cozens, J. (2001). Sickness absence in hospital physicians: 2 year follow up study on determinants. *Occupational and Environmental Medicine, 58,* 361–366.

Kropiunigg, U., Sebek, K., Leonhardsberger, A., Schemper, M., Dal-Bianco, P. (1999). Psychosocial risk factors for Alzheimer's disease. *Psychotherapy and Psychosomatic Medical Psychology 49*(5), 153–159.

Lewis, A. E. (1999). Reducing burnout: development of an oncology staff bereavement program. *Oncology Nursing Forum, 26,* 1065–1069.

Linn, M. W., Sandifer, R., Stein, S. (1985). Effects of unemployment on mental and physical health. *American Journal of Public Health 75,* 502–506.

Linton, S. J. (2001). Occupational psychological factors increase the risk for back pain: A systematic review. *Journal of Occupational Rehabilitation, 11*(1), 53–66.

Lundberg, U. (1999). Stress responses in low-status jobs and their relationships to health risks: musculoskeletal disorders. *Annals of New York Academy of Science, 896,* 162–172.

MacDonald, L. A., Karasek, R. A., Punnett, L., Scharf, T. (2001). Covariation between workplace physical and psychosocial stressors: evidence and implications for occupational health research and prevention. *Ergonomics, 44,* 696–718.

Maslach, C., Schaufeli, W. B., & Leiter, M. P. (2001). Job burnout. *Annual Review of Psychology, 52,* 397–422.

McDonough, P. (2000). Job insecurity and health. *International Journal of Health Services, 30,* 453–476.

Melamed, S., Yekutieli, D., Froom, P., Kristal-Bonch, E., & Ribak, J. (1999). Adverse work and environmental conditions predict occupational injuries. The Israeli Cardiovascular Occupational Risk Factors Determination in Israel (CORDIS) Study. *American Journal of Epidemiology, 150*(1), 18–26.

Norris, F. H., Matthews, B. A., Riad, J. K. (2000). Characterological, situational, and behavioral risk factors for motor vehicle accidents: A prospective examination. *Accidental Analysis and Prevention, 32,* 505–515.

Palmer, K. T., Walker-Bone, K., Griffin, M. J., Syddall, H., Pannett, B., Coggon, D., & Cooper, C. (2001). Prevalence and occupational associations of neck pain in the British population. *Scandanavian Journal of Work and Environmental Health, 27*(1), 49–56.

Parasuraman, S., & Purohit, Y. S. (2000). Distress and boredom among orchestra musicians: the two faces of stress. *Journal of Occupational Health Psychology, 5*(1), 74–83.

Parry-Jones, B., Grant, G., McGrath, M., Caldock, K., Ramcharan, P., & Robinson, C. A. (1998). Stress and job satisfaction among social workers, community nurses and community psychiatric nurses: implications for care management model. *Health and Social Care in the Community, 6,* 271–285.

Payne, N. (2001). Occupational stressors and coping as determinants of burnout in female hospice nurses. *Journal of Advanced Nursing, 33,* 396–405.

Piko, B. (1999). Work-related stress among nurses: A challenge for health care institutions. *Journal of Research in Society and Health, 119,* 156–162.

Rainey, D. W., & Hardy, L. (1999). Sources of stress, burnout and intention to terminate among rugby union referees. *Journal of Sports Science, 17,* 797–806.

Regehr, C., Hill, J., & Glancy, G. D. (2000). Individual predictors of traumatic reactions in firefighters. *Journal of Nervous and Mental Health Diseases, 188,* 333–339.

Reid, Y., Johnson, S., Morant, N., Kuipers, E., Szmukler, G., Thornicroft, G., Bebbington, P., & Prosser, D. (1999). Explanations for stress and satisfaction in mental health professionals: a qualitative study. *Social Psychiatry and Psychiatric Epidemiology* 34(6),301–308.

Rosch, P. (2002). Health and stress. [On-line]. Available at stress.org/problem.htm. Accessed 2/26/02.

Rout, U. R. (2000). Stress amongst district nurses: A preliminary investigation. *Journal of Clinical Nursing, 9,* 303–309.

Schaubroeck, J., Jones, J. R., & Xie, J. J. (2001). Individual differences in utilizing control to cope with job demands: Effects on susceptibility to infectious disease. *Journal of Applied Psychology, 86,* 265–278.

Severinsson, E. L., & Kamaker, D. (1999). Clinical nursing supervision in the workplace——Effects on moral stress and job satisfaction. *Journal of Nursing Management, 7*(2), 81–90.

Shigemi, J., Mino, Y., & Tsuda, T. (1999). The role of perceived job stress in the relationship between smoking and the development of peptic ulcers. *Journal of Epidemiology, 9,* 320–326.

Storr, C. L., Trinkoff, A. M., & Anthony, J. C. (1999). Job strain and non-medical drug use. *Drug and Alcohol Dependency, 55*(1–2), 45–51.

Taormina, R. J, & Law, C. M. (2000). Approaches to preventing burnout: The effects of personal stress management and organizational socialization. *Journal of Nursing Management, 8*(2), 89–99.

Teegen, F., & Muller, J. (2000). Trauma exposure and post-traumatic stress disorder in intensive care unit personnel. *Psychotherapy in Psychosomatic Medicine and Psychology, 50,* 384–390.

Thomas, S. (1993). *Women and anger.* New York: Springer.

2
Defining You:
How Assertive Are You?

I yam what I yam and dat's all what I yam.

—Popeye, The Sailor Man

This chapter provides information to help you define who you are and what you want. Without this kind of direction, it will be difficult to get to where you want to go.

McKay, Rogers, and McKay (1995) discussed one way of finding out who you are. When you were growing up, your parents probably never sat you down and told you who you were and how to get what you needed and wanted. You learned from watching them and imitating their behavior. You observed your parents' body language, tone of voice, choice of words and even choice of weapon when they were angry. You saw the results of not saying no, and may not have learned to ask for what you needed. You might have even have seen your parents show you how long-standing bitterness and anger resulted when problems were covered up instead of being resolved.

You probably also learned what anger felt like and how scary it could be. Because you depended on your parents for everything, in your eyes they were all-powerful and all-knowing. You needed your parents' acceptance and approval and you needed to find a way to deal with their anger.

You may have learned to deny your feelings and needs in order to feel safe and wanted, acting compliant and always/ ready to please. Choosing this route can lead to being passive or passive-aggressive as an adult. You may have learned to be just as aggressive as one of your parents and that may have become your way of coping with anger and feeling safe. Neither the passive nor the aggressive style of relating works for long and you probably won't get your needs met that way, either.

29

Suppose your supervisor arrives late for an appointment with you. You wait and wait. You drink several cups of coffee and you fume. Then you begin to worry that something bad may have happened to her. She finally breezes in, apologizing and telling you all the things that went wrong for her so far today. The more your supervisor talks, the angrier you get. You're so mad at her that you don't know what to do.

Let's take a look at what's going on here. What is the stress that can trigger anger and blame? One stressful thing about this situation is that your supervisor shows she doesn't care about anything but herself. The stress of this situation can trigger blaming thoughts, such as, My supervisor is on a selfish talkathon and doesn't care one iota about me or my problems and doesn't even respect me enough to come on time.

If you want to empower yourself, you will have to begin to look at this situation as one in which your supervisor has a need to be listened to and that she came late because she had other needs that took priority over meeting with you. If you want to give up your anger, you have to give up your expectation that your supervisor will be on time and will listen to you. Once you do that, anger and blame fall away.

What can you do instead to ensure you won't get into anger and blaming in the future?

1. Decide if you want to confront your supervisor about her lateness. Is it worth it to you to have the problem out in the open or will it make your job even more unbearable? Consult with a colleague about how she'd handle the situation in an assertive way.

2. If you're worried about your supervisor being late, arrange to pick her up in plenty of time to make your meeting.

3. If it bothers you to wait for your supervisor, bring a book or complete some other work that needs to be done while you wait.

4. Realize that your supervisor probably isn't going to change the way she talks. If you want to share, you're going to have to find a polite way to interrupt, such as, "I have something to say on that point" or "That reminds me, I have an idea I want to share."

Your turn. Write down a situation that occurred in which you felt angry and wanted to blame the other person. Write down the particulars of the situation here:

Write down what triggered stress in you:

What were your thoughts urging you to blame the other person?

Write down at least three options you have to prevent this situation from happening in the future:

1.

2.

3.

Write down a date when you plan to implement at least one of these options:

Write down what happened when you implemented one of these options:

Decide if this was a good option for you. If it wasn't, choose another option and try that. Report your findings:

SAYING GOOD-BYE TO OLD ABUSES

Before you can define what you want and what will be empowering, you need to release from your mind/body/spirit childhood feelings of abuse and neglect. This will allow you to value yourself (Mellody & Miller, 1989) and decide on your path to empowerment. Many of us have experienced emotional, physical, or sexual abuse. Even verbal criticism, put-downs and unfair accusations are considered abuse. Use Exercise 11 to assist you in this process.

EXERCISE 11 Releasing Childhood Abuse/Neglect

Directions: Go through all the abusive or neglectful experiences you've had, including physical (hitting, shoving, pinching, not being fed, clothed, held, or protected); intellectual (derogatory comments about your abilities, no acknowledgment at all); emotional (tried to stop you from expressing your feelings or from crying, no response to feelings or crying); sexual (touched you sexually or made you report your sexual experiences, no response to report of sexual abuse/neglect); spiritual and ethical (accused you unfairly of wrongdoing without apologizing; never provided spiritual or ethical information).

For each instance, write down the type of abuse or neglect, the person's name, your age, what exactly happened, how you felt then, and how you feel now.

(continued)

EXERCISE 11 (*continued*)

Abuse Type	Abuser	Your Age	The Details	Feelings Then	Feelings Now

Look back at each situation, especially the column "how you feel now." If you feel comfortable when you think about each situation, read on in this book. For each situation that you don't feel comfortable about, complete one or more of the following procedures:

1. Close your eyes and make the feeling a color. Turn the color into a liquid. Picture it flowing out of you and going far away, somewhere where it can no longer influence you.

2. Write the following affirmation on a 3 x 5 card and read it at least 20 times a day: This feeling is from the past. It no longer exists. It no longer has any hold over me.

BECOMING ASSERTIVE

Finding out who you are and becoming who you want to be will continue until the day you die. You will always be discovering new and uncharted aspects of yourself. To start you on that voyage, if you haven't made many inroads, this section can help you accept your abilities and self-worth, investigate your rights, identify your fears and find alternatives, assess your assertive skills, challenge your "shoulds," identify your real and ideal self, set realistic goals, identify expectations, make a contract to change, use "I" messages, and stick to the point.

Accept Your Abilities and Self-Worth

As mentioned earlier, low self-esteem frequently leads to feeling disempowered. Use Exercise 12 to enhance your self-esteem.

EXERCISE 12 I Am Strong and Self-Confident

Directions: Say or read the following meditation at least once a day. If you prefer, read it into a tape recorder and listen to the results daily.

I now declare the past over and done. It no longer exists. It has returned to the nothingness from which it arose. Now that it is over, I am free. Now that it is over, I have a new sense of pride and self-worth. I have a new sense of confidence in my abilities to love and support myself. Each day it becomes clearer and clearer that I am capable of positive growth and change. I am strong and growing stronger every day. I am one with all life. I am one with the Universal power and intelligence (or God). Divine wisdom leads me and guides me every minute, every hour,

(continued)

EXERCISE 12 (*continued*)

every day. I am completely safe and secure, moving forward to my highest good. I do this with total joy and ease. I am becoming a new person, living in a world of my choosing that is exactly perfect for me. I am deeply grateful for everything I am and everything I have. I am prosperous and blessed, in perfect harmony with everything and everyone around me. All is well and continues to be well in my world.

Claim Your Rights

Part of finding out who you are is affirming your rights as a person. The following rights are yours, no matter what anyone tells you.

- You have the right to judge your own behavior, thoughts and feelings and to take responsibility for their initiation and consequences.
- You have the right to choose not to give reasons or excuses for your behavior.
- You have the right to change your mind.
- You have the right to make excuses and take the consequences.
- You have the right to say, "I don't know."
- You have the right to say no without feeling guilty.
- You have the right to find dignity in self-expression and self-enhancement through your work.
- You have the right to be recognized for your contribution by being provided with an environment within which your skills are utilized and proper rewards are offered.
- You have the right to work in an environment that is physically, emotionally and spiritually healthy.
- You have the right to participate in policies that affect your work.
- You have the right to take social and political action to enhance your work situation and consumer treatment.

Use Exercise 13 to identify your rights.

EXERCISE 13 Your Rights

Directions: Take a look at the rights listed above. Which ones seem most acceptable to you? Which ones don't? Pick one right you find the most difficult to accept. Write a paragraph describing why it is difficult. Then write a paragraph describing why you can accept it. If all the rights seem valid to you, write at least one other right that you perceive to be yours.

A right that seems the most the difficult to accept is . . .

This right is difficult to accept because . . .

Now that I think about it, I am beginning to accept this right because . . .

Another right that is mine is . . .

Identify Your Fears

Although it may seem like a wonderful change to be empowered, fears may be keeping you from reaching your full potential. Common fears that could be preventing your empowerment include fear that you will be rejected if you change, will be unable to function appropriately in a new role, won't be able to control your emotions, or will lose old protective devices. Other fears include fear of learning the "truth" about yourself, fear of being retaliated against, and fear of being punished by authority figures.

You may even have a fear of success, which can occur if success means other challenges and changes. If you *are* successful, it could mean having to contend with competitive feelings and behavior from others, isolation from peers, and other complex problems.

Another common fear is the fear of anger. If you have this fear, you may assume that if you express your feelings you might lose control, which means different things to different people. Your interpretation is probably based on early family experiences, where the appropriate expression of anger was learned. You may interpret an angry tone of voice as losing control, or throwing an object, or even blowing up in exasperation. Fear of your own anger and its effects on others can prevent you from even experimenting with the expression of anger, thinking that such expression may devastate others. This kind of fear is common if you've had little experience expressing your anger or have received negative reactions from others when they have dared to express their feelings. This fear can lead to vacillation between acquiescence (until feelings build up) and aggression (where a small incident sets off an outburst), followed by guilt feelings (especially if you've been reprimanded for past expressions of anger). This self-enforcing syndrome can become a never-ending cycle unless assertiveness intervenes.

You may also fear being assertive because you think others might confront you about your behavior. This could happen, but assertive training will help you deal constructively with these situations. The irrational component of this fear is that confrontation will lead to learning "bad" things about yourself. Most of the time, confrontation leads to learning about both your strengths and limitations. Once limitations are pinpointed, they can be worked on.

Fear of being retaliated against is also a common fear. If you hold this attitude you fear that others will retaliate against you for being assertive. The fact is, reasonable people will be more accepting of assertive behavior, not less. Aggression or acquiescence are more likely to be met with retaliation.

Fear of punishment is usually a carryover from childhood. When you were a child, you were responsible to your parents and your small stature and limited repertoire of interpersonal skills did place you at the mercy of these authority figures. You probably have vivid memories of being punished legitimately and illegitimately by your mother or father. Holding this childhood view of authority figures and attributing unlimited power and punishment rights to supervisors or administrators exemplifies a developmental arrest in relation to authority figures. Assertive training can help you examine your myths and childhood perceptions in light of being adult. Use Exercise 14 to help you identify fears that may be hindering your assertiveness.

EXERCISE 14 Fears That Hinder My Assertiveness

Directions: People learn to be nonassertive. You can become more aware of which fears hinder your assertiveness by looking at the following list. For each one that applies to you, think of a situation that resulted in being inhibited by your fear.

1. Fear of being rejected. Example:

2. Fear of being too aggressive. Example:

3. Fear of being unfeminine or unmasculine. Example:

4. Fear of losing familiar coping devices. Example:

5. Fear of losing control. Example:

6. Fear of learning the "truth" about myself. Example:

7. Fear of being retaliated against. Example:

(*continued*)

EXERCISE 14 (*continued*)

8. Fear of being punished by authority figures. Example:

9. Fear of _____. Example:

Be Assertive, Not Fearful

Now that you've identified and specified your fears, you are in a better position to examine them and find a better response. Many times unrealistic expectation, including fear of success, can keep you from acting because you assume there will be dire consequences if you act assertively. Ask yourself, What is the worst thing that could happen if I assert myself about this? Concretize your fears. Write them down and examine them in the clear light of day. How likely is that to happen? So what if it does? You're up to handling it if it does. You're strong and tough.

You can't always count on someone else to provide support for you if you choose to be assertive. Be prepared. Write down a message you can give yourself that will help you to be more assertive:

Be sure to carry this message with you and use it when the crucial moment comes to be assertive.

Examine your expectations about being assertive and take them to their ultimate conclusion. This kind of exercise can often provide you with the courage to act assertively, because you will begin to realize that you can handle even your most feared situation. Use Exercise 15 to work toward reducing your fears and empowering yourself.

EXERCISE 15 Finding a Better Response Than Fear

Directions: Examine your unrealistic expectations by filling in the answers to the following statements.

What is the worse thing that could happen if I assert myself?

If this occurs, I can deal with this by:

If that doesn't work, I can:

Even if my worst fears come true, I can:

If I become successful and empowered, I can handle it by:

Identify Your Real and Your Ideal Self

Pressures to conform, to be less assertive, and to be less of who you really are come from colleagues, administrators, families, and friends. Receiving one message in words and another through action can lead to ambivalence and confusion. In a situation like this, you may vacillate between seeking support or solace from peers and talking about or deriding them with others. This kind of vacillation is counterproductive because it leads to divisiveness and funnels energy that could be used to achieve goals. This is why it's important to identify your real and your ideal self. Take a look at Exercise 16 now.

EXERCISE 16 Your Real and Your Ideal Self

Directions: Empowered, assertive people take stock of who they are before taking steps to change unwanted behaviors. Take some time to describe who you are and how you would like to be different. This is an assessment of your real and your ideal self. There is space for you to write "shoulds" that seem to be keeping you from being who you want to be, for example, "I should be nice," or "I should only do what other people tell me," or "I should go along with the crowd."

Real self: I am a person who

1.
2.
3.
4.
5.
6.
7.

Ideal self: I would like to be more

1.
2.
3.
4.
5.
6.
7.

"Shoulds" that prevent me from being my ideal self are

1.
2.
3.
4.
5.
6.
7.

Feeling powerless about your ability to control what happens to you can result in statements such as "Things can't be changed" or "What can I do? I'm only one person." This type of pseudo-innocence negates your real power and so does using "feminine wiles," that is, deferring to others, hesitating, apologizing unnecessarily, or disparaging your own viewpoint. This makes a woman look indecisive and disempowered. Sometimes just holding the thought that you do have power can provide the needed extra boost to move toward empowerment.

Women often have characteristics that make them especially susceptible to disempowerment. They are more likely to be called by their first names, especially if they do not hold a title such as doctor or professor, although that does not always protect them. Also, women tend to reveal more of themselves in conversation, and this tendency toward self-disclosure places them in a more vulnerable position than men who withhold such information. Nonverbal behaviors women are apt to learn are to smile, not to swear or raise their voices, to touch others and be touched, to avert their eyes when confronted, and to be especially careful about their appearance. This essential early learning can lead to men who perform and women who attract. One of the ways that women can begin to reverse these learned stances of male-female relationships is to practice reversing verbal and nonverbal components that enhance their personal power and effectiveness. Training in assertiveness can promote this practice.

Educational experiences can also reinforce passive behavior. Most students are not taught assertive skills and are often told they are being taught to be independent, but are given little responsibility prior to graduation. At the same time, students who are overly inquisitive or who challenge their teachers are labeled as troublemakers or are given messages that they had better conform in order to receive approval or grades. Then they are expected (magically) to be self-directed and independent at the moment of graduation without any prior practice. Much of this may be because many teachers are not assertive themselves and so are not role models for assertiveness, nor are they able to teach students how to be assertive. Without effective role models or practice, you can't expect to be assertive unless you undergo additional learning experiences.

There is more to this equation. Many work sites have written rules that they want their employees to be proactive and creative in their response to problem situations. Unwritten rules often hinder assertiveness. This can lead to aggressive administrators who join forces with nonassertive employees to undermine employees who are assertive. If you work in a setting in which you know you cannot count on your peers for support when you're under fire, you'll be less likely to take an assertive stances. If you're a woman, you may have difficulty in leadership positions because other women may not view you as an authority figure. Female subordinates may mistrust your word and be more critical of your personal style than of a male leader's, who is judged on effectiveness. These expectations must come from early family experiences, where the mother was nurturing and expressive and the father was the breadwinner. For this reasons, female leaders who are supportive, expressive, and nurturing may be more accepted as leaders than those who want to complete tasks, coordinate others' work, and solve problems. The result of this conditioning is that female leaders may be in continual conflict about whether they should be nurturing or assertive.

Men can have just as many problems with assertiveness. Many of them learn to cover over their inadequate feelings by being aggressive or by railroading other people into doing what they want, by refusing to commit to a relationship, or by being indirect. Some men are just shy and avoid any confrontation.

INTERPERSONAL EMPOWERMENT

Could your relationships with others be hindering your empowerment? Find out by going to Exercise 17 now.

EXERCISE 17 Could Your Relationships Be Hindering Your Empowerment?

Directions: Circle YES or NO in answer to the questions below to find out how your relationships with other people may be interfering with your ability to feel empowered. The more YES answers you've circled, the more relationships may be hindering your empowerment.

1. My supervisor is not supportive of my efforts to feel
   or act empowered.   YES NO
2. Colleagues tease or scold me about my efforts to feel
   or act empowered.   YES NO
3. My supervisor teases me or disrespects my efforts
   to feel or act empowered.   YES NO
4. I resent at least one past or current relationship.   YES NO
5. I have at least one person I must deal with at work
   who is difficult.   YES NO
6. At least person in my life does not hear me when I try
   to tell him or her something.   YES NO

No matter how hard you work to empower yourself, it's going to be difficult to achieve if the important people in your life sabotage you. What words can you use to convince family, friends, coworkers or supervisors to support you and empower you? Let's take a look at some statements you could use to gain their support.

- "I'm working to change _____ [your behavior] and I could really use your help. "Would you be willing to help me by _____ [their behavior] and by _____ [your behavior]?"
- "It would be helpful if you'd _____ [their behavior]. Can I count on you?"

Use your responses to the above three statements to set goals for following:

1. Who you will talk to about these matters (make a list of their names here):

2. When you will talk to each person (list the dates and names here):

Another way to get your partner, family, colleagues, or friends to be more supportive of your efforts to solve relationship problems is to call a meeting and ask each person for support. Scheduling a meeting is a good way to work out difficulties with other people in your life. Settle on a day and time that works for the majority. Convince them how important this is to you. (You might have to convince yourself first by giving yourself permission to be the center of everyone's focus. Go ahead. You deserve it!) At first some of them may grumble, make excuses and not want to come to your meeting. Be persistent. Reassure them that they can get something out of this, too. Ask them to write down one thing they'd like to change about their relationship with you and to bring it to the meeting. Promise that their concerns will be brought up at the meeting and that you'll support their right to find a solution if they will help you solve your problem. When the meeting takes place, ask everyone to write down on a small card or piece of paper the one thing each wants to see change. Collect their wishes and add them with yours to a pot or hat. Draw one wish out at a time and spend 10 to 15 minutes per person discussing that person's wish and how to achieve it. Tell the group that everybody gets to speak, but one at a time, and no arguing. Pick out another wish and repeat the process until everyone's problem has been discussed and each person (including you) has at least one possible solution to the problem. If this kind of meeting seems too much for you to handle, take an assertiveness class to help raise your confidence.

You can't change your biological family, but if your family members aren't providing the solace and support you need, be assertive, find your own group of like-minded people. Connect with them, spend time with them, and find support for you and your ideas with them. That will make it easier to be with your biological family and can reduce tension: You won't expect so much from family members anymore because you will have another source of support.

Challenge Counterproductive Beliefs

Although it is admirable to strive to handle situations well, it is counterproductive to expect yourself to change old patterns overnight when you've spent years developing them. You know that some beliefs held by others will end up defeating your attempts to be assertive unless you prepare for them. The following are some beliefs you especially need to consider and prepare for:

• *Isn't assertiveness just a way of manipulating others to get what you want?* No. Being assertive means standing up for your rights, knowing full well that others have rights, too. Being assertive is less manipulative than verbal stabs in the back, avoiding important issues, or blowing up.
• *If someone gets angry because I'm assertive, isn't that anger my fault?* No. You cannot be responsible for another's behavior, but you might be able to teach that person how to accept reasonable limits without becoming unduly angry.
• *Shouldn't I be able to meet other people's demands and needs?* No. It's impossible to be all things to all people. You have a right to assert your own needs, too. Allowing someone to hurt or drain you is not constructive to either of you.
• *Shouldn't I be able to think spontaneously of the perfect response in every situation?* Assertiveness is a skill that requires planning, practice, and hard work to master. To expect yourself to handle situations in a new way spontaneously is unrealistic and

will lead to frustration. This can cause you to downplay your potential. Second, you cannot be responsible for anyone else's reactions and feelings—only your own. One risk you take when asserting yourself is that others may not like what you do or say, but it's a risk you can learn to handle.

Being assertive means being able to admit to both strengths and limitations. Being able to say "I don't know" is a human, assertive response.

It's important to separate out which issue in assertiveness is whose. Don't expect others to promise *before* you assert yourself that they will not react negatively. That is not an assertive act, it's a controlling act. Daring to be assertive means taking the risk that others may not agree or feel comfortable with your behavior.

• *Shouldn't I be able to be assertive without ever threatening or frustrating others?* You may be worried that being assertive will threaten your relationship with the other person. It's doubtful the other person is so fragile that your words could produce irreparable harm. It is true that if you are assertive, other people may view your behavior as a threat. You have a 50-50 chance either way. You need to ask yourself whether being liked is a useful goal. Chances are quite good that regardless of what others do, you will like yourself better if you assert yourself. Even if the other person gets angry if you assert yourself, you can handle it. Besides, if that person becomes unreasonably angry, it's doubtful the situation will turn out badly unless you resort to aggressiveness and attack in response to that anger. Remember, the other person has to take responsibility for his or her own anger because you can't.

On the other hand, remaining silent and hoping that more appropriate leadership will occur is an avoidance of responsibility. For example, by remaining silent and allowing yourself to participate in ineffective work groups, you negate your potential as an informal leader with that group. By using assertive behavior you could exert important leadership in those situations. You must have met people who have little formal authority, but who are able to influence others by the sheer power of their personality or actions. This is an example of how informal leadership works.

• *Shouldn't I handle situations better than I do?* Putting yourself down for not handling situations as well as you would like is a waste of time. If you think of a better response afterwards, write it down and use it later. As long as you and the other person are alive, situations can continue to be resolved. If you wake up at 3 a.m. with an idea for how you could have been assertive in a situation, get up and write your thoughts. Then when you are ready, approach the other person with a comment such as, "I've been thinking about our argument last week and I'd like to talk about it and resolve it," or "Remember that disagreement we had yesterday. I'd like to talk to you about it."

• *Won't people think I'm cold and uncaring if I assert myself?* You may be accused of being cold or uncaring by people who try to manipulate you to comply with what they want. Taking care of others all the time and not allowing them or you to relate as equals leads to a parent–child relationship, not an adult–adult relationships. Treating others as capable people who can act independently will enrich a relationship.

• *Can I become so assertive that I overwhelm other people?* You cannot be too assertive. One aspect of assertiveness is that it's appropriate to the situation.

Differentiate Assertiveness From Aggression and Avoidance

Before you assess your level of assertiveness, it's important to be able to tell the difference between assertiveness, aggressiveness, and avoiding or passive-aggressive behavior. *Aggressive* and *avoiding behavior* are similar in one way: both are the opposite of assertiveness.

When you use aggressive or avoiding behavior, you allow someone else to define you and your rights. This can lead to feelings of inadequacy and insecurity. Hurts are turned inward and depression, self-blame, self-punishment, and resentment develop.

Note that anger is not aggression. Anger is a legitimate feeling that can be expressed passively, assertively, or aggressively. If not expressed, it can fester inside and lead to physical illness. If expressed aggressively, it can get you in trouble or lead to feelings of guilt.

When you avoid dealing with an issue or acquiesce and take the path of least resistance, you allow others to choose for you, decide for you, and speak for you. "Don't rock the boat!" is your motto. This can lead to feeling defensive, guilty, and fearful. You're more apt to back down under fire. When you are so fearful of confrontation and conflict, you are the first to smooth things over before taking time to examine the issues involved. When you are avoidant or acquiescent, you are apt to turn to others for answers, are reactive rather than problem solving, and apt to exhibit hostile or aggressive behavior.

This pattern can emerge in overt or subtle forms. Acquiescent and aggressive behaviors are two sides of the same coin. Both are reactive rather than goal-direct or proactive. Both reflect underlying insecurity, represent indirect communication, and demonstrate a lack of taking responsibility for your own actions and feelings.

The main problem with remaining acquiescent is that anger gradually builds up. Resentful feelings can then erupt in emotional upset, outbursts, or passive-aggressive acts. The hidden aggressive component of acquiescent behavior usually can be noted in an interchange by the other party who often senses a lack of respect and experiences pain or decreased learning. When you acquiesce, you may humiliate or prevent the other person from accomplishing a goal due to procrastination or passive resistance. You also act as a role model, showing others how to remain dependent rather than being independent and empowered. When you acquiesce, others may sense restrictive and subtle hostility in the form of nagging, or they may detect the subtle put-down message when you daydream in response to an enthusiastic and assertive presentation.

It is difficult to see the line between hidden aggressions and avoiding or acquiescent behaviors. At times, avoiding behaviors have elements of aggressiveness. For example, calling in sick due to a headache or diarrhea on an especially busy day may be a way of punishing yourself, but it can also "get back at" others by forcing them to cope with a difficult situation without you. Table 2.1 shows some hidden aggressions and avoiding behaviors.

Assertive Responses

It's not unusual to confuse assertiveness with aggressiveness. Let's take a look at some assertive responses.

Situation 1: You approach a colleague about an error she made. As you begin to talk to her, she accuses you of picking on her. An assertive response would be, "Let's talk this over and straighten this out."

Situation 2: You and a colleague agreed he would complete his portion of the job for a meeting that is to take place that afternoon. You realize he has not given you the report yet. An assertive comment to make to him is, "We agreed your report would be available today."

Situation 3: Someone comes up to you while you are in the middle of an important task and asks you for help with a less

TABLE 2.1 Hidden Aggressions and Avoidant/Acquiescent Behavior

Types	Examples
Chronic forgetfulness	"Forgetting" to complete an important task. Delaying helping someone who asks for help.
Breaking confidentiality	Sharing private information with a third person without first checking if it's okay.
Procrastinating	Always finding something else to do besides completing the agreed upon task.
Overhelpful/stifling	Not allowing others to be independent; the let-me-do-that-for-you syndrome.
Nagging	"Haven't you finished that yet?" "You are going to finish it, aren't you?"
Somatization/withdrawal	Calling in sick with a headache, backache, or diarrhea before an important meeting, class, appointment, etc.
Wish to escape	Fantasizing, daydreaming, or changing the subject when a confrontation is about to occur.
Guilt induction	Chiding others, hoping to coerce them into doing what you want them to do under the guise of being helpful or diligent; statements often contain the word "should," e.g., "You should . . ."
Unfair criticism	Statements comparing others in an unfavorable light, e.g., "Gaining weight, aren't you?" and "I don't see what's taking so long. [Name of another person] would have been able to do this much better [quicker, cheaper, etc.].
Teasing	"Oh, come on, don't be so serious."
Passive resistance	Saying yes or agreeing to do a task, but never acting; the verbal stab in the back.
Intimidation through dependency	Speaking so softly or appearing so fragile that the other person is intimidated.
Over-agreeableness	Agreeing with everything and anything so as not to rock the boat.

important task. An assertive comment would be, "I'm just finishing this up. I can help you in 10 minutes."

Situation 4: Your boss catches an error you made and tells you about it. An assertive response is, "You're right. I did make a mistake."

Situation 5: Someone you know starts to holler and berate you. An assertive response is, "I don't like to be shouted at, but I'd like to hear about what's upsetting you."

Situation 6: A family member is always signing you up for courses and meetings you have no interest in. An assertive response is, "I appreciate your concern, but I want to make my own decisions."

COMPONENTS OF ASSERTIVE BEHAVIOR

Presentation of Self

Now it's your turn to look at your assertive skills and see what behaviors you might want to change. Be aware that no one is totally assertive at all times in all situations. You may be assertive at work but have a tough time saying no to your partner or child or vice versa.

One component of assessing assertiveness is the presentation of yourself. The question to be asked is, How do I present myself to others? Do I look and sound assertive, aggressive, or avoiding? This component includes verbal and nonverbal aspects.

Nonverbal Aspects of Assertiveness

Some nonverbal areas to assess are speaking in a loud enough, firm, fluent voice; maintaining eye contact; and using appropriate facial expressions, gestures, body postures, and positioning. No matter how clear your message, you will appear unsure of yourself if you don't look the person in the eye when speaking. This holds true for most cultural situations. There are a few specific exceptions in which eye contact without touching may create anxiety in the other person. If you don't speak loudly enough to be heard easily, the other person will likely think you aren't serious about what you're saying. Likewise, if you have a frozen smile on your face when discussing a serious topic, or wave your arms wildly when trying to make a point, others will not see you as an assertive person. In the first situation, they will not know why you are smiling or will be confused about whether or not to take you seriously. In the second situation, the observer will tend to get carried away watching your gestures and may miss many of your words. A relaxed body posture conveys self-confidence, interest, openness, and nondefensiveness.

Facing the person to whom you are speaking is part of an assertive presentation of self. Make sure you stand or sit an appropriate distance from the other person, being aware this distance may vary by cultural, institutional, professional, or interpersonal rules. Observe assertive people in a similar situation and copy their performance.

Verbal Aspects of Assertiveness

Some verbal areas to assess are initiating and maintaining conversations; expressing thoughts, feelings, and expectations in a clear, concise way; stating and staying with the problem or issue at hand; and using "I" messages. Often, you may not be the one to begin the conversation, but if the issue is important to you, it would be an assertive move to try to maintain the conversation on the agreed-upon topic. Others may try to end the conversation and cut off communication, but you can learn how to increase the possibility for ongoing communication.

Persistence is an important aspect of assertiveness. If you state your point or feeling in a clear, concise way, you are less likely to be misunderstood, and you will allow more time for others to speak. When you make long-winded or unrelated comments, you tend to lose your listener and will not be viewed as serious or assertive. Sticking to the issue at hand may be difficult for you, but it is something you can learn to do through practice and diligence.

"I" messages are another important aspect of assertiveness. "I" messages convey that you take responsibility for what you think, feel, or want. Some examples of assertive "I" messages are "I think that's a fine idea," "I feel upset about this," "I want to focus on working this out," or "This is an issue I can't compromise on." Some messages that masquerade as "I" messages are "I think you feel . . .," or "I feel you ought to . . .," or "I want you to . . .". In the first set of authentic and empowering messages, you take responsibility for your own thoughts, feelings, desires, or actions. In the second set of inauthentic "I" messages, you try to take responsibility for the other person by pretending to know what the other person thinks or feels.

Certain "we" messages can also be assertive. Don't confuse "we" collaborative messages with "we" undifferentiated ones. In the collaborative statement, the message is "Let's work on this together, we each have the skill, energy and responsibility to do this." In the undifferentiated statement, such as "Let's take our bath now," the message is "It's your bath, but I don't have a clear identity or plan, and besides, you need to be treated like an infant and cajoled or tricked." Undifferentiated messages are nonassertive while collaborative messages are assertive. Examples of "we" assertive messages are, "Let's talk this over and find a compromise," "I think we can work this out," or "Let's work together."

Another type of statement you will find useful to delete from your assertive repertoire is the manipulative *why* question. Phrasing a statement in a *why* format evades taking responsibility for the question. Many times the person who asks such a question already knows the answer. For example, the question, "Why didn't you finish yet?" really means "I think you should have finished." To be more assertive, limit or delete the use of "Why didn't you? . . .", "Why don't you? . . .", and "Why can't you? . . .".

Some other nonassertive behaviors in the presentation of self are repeating unnecessary words; pausing too often; seeming to be speechless; stumbling or stammering when speaking; laughing nervously; looking up, down, or away from the person with whom you're speaking; looking angry when saying you're not; saying you are angry and not looking it; smiling when expressing anger, disagreement, grief, or seriousness; not speaking loudly enough or firmly enough; speaking too loudly; standing or sitting too close to or too far away from your listener; over-apologizing for or over-explaining an issue, your opinion, or your behavior; getting sidetracked onto irrelevant topics; talking too much and not allowing others to state their views; using sarcasm, whining, pleading, cajoling, guilt induction, sighing or rolling your eyes; qualifying your statements with comments such as, "I'm sorry, but . . .," "This probably isn't right, but . . .," "This may be a dumb question, but . . .," and using "you" or blaming messages.

"You" or blaming statements are apt to put others on the defensive. Their message is "You shouldn't have done that," or "It's all your fault."

"You" statements attack the other person. There is no attempt on your part to state how you feel or to take responsibility for your share of the situation. A variation of the blaming statement is, "Why didn't you . . . ?" or "Why don't you . . . ?" Here the message is, "If you were smarter, you would have" or "Since you can't figure it out for yourself, I'll tell you what to do." This is not to suggest that you banish the words *you* or *why* from your vocabulary. In fact, some assertive statements do contain why and you, such as "Why don't you and I talk this over?" or "I wonder why that happened?" or "What's your view of why we're deadlocked?" and "I want to thank you for your help."

Active Orientation

Another component of assertiveness is an active orientation to life. You don't wait for situations to improve, you take action to improve them. You put forth policies, procedures, and solutions. You can work toward full capacity in a self-directed way. You tell others what you expect and what others can expect from you. Other aspects of this component include reminding others of deadlines or time frames within which tasks must be completed, telling others about special skills or achievements, and planning and working toward long- and short-term goals.

Part of setting goals is examining realistic and unrealistic work objectives. Unrealistic work objectives include

- the need to be needed
- the need to be liked
- the need to master impossible tasks or impossible situations
- the need to be the "good child" by winning approval
- the need to have others feel sorry for you

Realistic work goals include

- making money
- earning a living
- pursuing glory, status or prestige
- being rewarded for interest or skill
- doing meaningful work
- personal growth and change

Constructive Work Habits

Constructive work habits comprise another component of assertiveness. This component includes structuring a satisfying day, setting limits on others' interruptions and requests, concentrating on one task at a time, completing unpleasant tasks without procrastinating, and structuring work to reward yourself.

Giving and Taking Criticism

Giving and taking criticism, evaluation, and help is another component of assertiveness. Aspects of this component include feeling comfortable taking compliments, praising others, owning up to your mistakes or errors, pointing out others' limitations or need for learning, asking for assistance when you need it, and remaining calm while being observed or evaluated.

Controlling Anxiety and Fear

A final component of assertiveness is the ability to control anxiety and fear. Some indicators of this aspect are a sense of comfort when standing up for your rights, disagreeing with others, expressing anger, hearing others' anger, handling a put-down or being teased, asking for legitimate limits to your workload, and taking a reasonable risk.

Assertive Assessment

Now that you know about all the aspects of assertiveness, it's time to put them all together. See Exercise 18 and assess your assertiveness level.

EXERCISE 18 Assertiveness Assessment

Directions: Use this exercise to assess your current assertiveness level. The items running down the left side of the page refer to the five components of assertive behavior: presentation of self; active work orientation, constructive work habits; giving and taking criticism, evaluation, and help; and control of anxiety or fear. There are several indicators for each component. The columns that run across the top of the assessment refer to people with whom you find it relatively easy or difficult to be assertive. Ignore the spaces that don't apply to you. Remember: No one is assertive all the time. Use *U* for usually, *F* for frequently or *S* for seldom.

	Interpersonal situations	
	With one	In a
Behaviors	person*	group
Presentation of Self		
Verbal components		
I make clear, concise statements	——	——
I stick to the issue/problem at hand	——	——
I can initiate and maintain a conversation	——	——

*You may wish to identify specific people you have difficulty being assertive with and see if you always have a problem being assertive with your boss, partner, children, relatives, a specific friend, a supervisee, a teacher, a physician, a police officer, a sales clerk, or others. Devote special attention to those areas where you wrote an *S*. Note that you probably lack assertive skills in these areas. Regardless of the results of this ̄ssment, you may choose not to change your behavior. It's all up to you!

(continued)

EXERCISE 18 (*continued*)

Behaviors	Interpersonal situations	
	With one person*	In a group
I express my thoughts and feelings openly	___	___
I use "I" or collaborative "we" statements	___	___
Nonverbal components		
I speak in a loud, firm, fluent voice	___	___
I maintain eye contact	___	___
My facial expression is appropriate to my words	___	___
My body posture conveys interest and openness	___	___
I position myself to sit or stand an appropriate distance from others	___	___
Active orientation		
I suggest new policies, procedures, and solutions	___	___
I work to my full capacity in a self-directed way	___	___
I tell others exactly what they can expect from me	___	___
I ask others exactly what they expect of me	___	___
I plan short-term and long-term goals	___	___
I work to achieve my goals	___	___
I tell others of my special skills and achievements	___	___
I remind others of deadlines or time frames without nagging or trying to make them feel guilty	___	___
Constructive work habits		
I structure my day so I am reasonably satisfied with its outcomes	___	___
I limit other people's interruptions	___	___
I concentrate on one task at a time	___	___
I find a way to complete unpleasant tasks	___	___
I say no to illegitimate requests	___	___
I structure my work to reward myself	___	___
Giving and taking criticism and help		
I can take compliments and feel comfortable	___	___
I can praise others for their achievements	___	___
I own up to my mistakes and limitations	___	___
I point out others' limitations or need for learning in a neutral way	___	___
I ask for assistance when I need it	___	___
I remain calm when I'm being observed or evaluated	___	___
Control of anxiety or fear		
I can feel comfortable when		
Standing up for my rights	___	___
Disagreeing	___	___

(*continued*)

EXERCISE 18 (*continued*)

Behaviors	Interpersonal situations	
	With one person*	In a group
Expressing anger	——	——
Dealing with others' anger	——	——
Handling a put-down or teasing	——	——
Asking for a legitimate limit to my workload	——	——
Taking a reasonable risk	——	——

SET ASSERTIVENESS GOALS

If you do decide to change to more assertive behaviors, the first step is to prioritize your assertiveness needs. Look back at Exercise 18. Mark the items you want to work on. You will be setting goals related to those items. Go back and rank them in order of priority from most difficult (last) to easiest to accomplish (1). Remember to start with your number 1 in order to build in success.

Choose a Simple Two-Person Situation to Start

In general, it is more difficult to establish new behavior in a complex situation (where more than 2 people are involved) in which you are taken by surprise (have to think on your feet). It is also difficult to change behavior in an ongoing relationship that tests you to the limit, probably because you have a history with that person and each time you see him or her, you are reminded of past encounters.

Choose a simple, two–person situation to start with. You want to build in success. Make sure the situation doesn't have a long history of negative outcome and will have no effect on important people or things in your life. For example, don't pick a situation in which you must confront your boss as one of your first goals. Work up to that with simpler, circumscribed situations such as saying no to a stranger or to the clerk behind the counter of a deli you frequent, or asking for help from a doorman or salesperson. Prior to setting an assertiveness goal, complete Exercise 19, "Breaking Chain Reactions."

EXERCISE 19 Breaking Chain Reactions

Directions: This exercise was devised to help you begin to break habitual responses that decrease your assertiveness and disempower you.

1. Describe three situations in which you have an habitual nonassertive response.

   Situation 1:

   Situation 2:

   Situation 3:

2. Write your usual response to each situation.

   Situation 1:

   Situation 2:

(*continued*)

EXERCISE 19 (*continued*)

Situation 3:

3. Pretend that you paused and *instead* of giving your habitual response, you decided to try something different. Write that response.

   A new response to situation 1 is:

   A new response to situation 2 is:

   A new response to situation 3 is:

4. Try out your new response to one of the situations by role-playing it, and then by using it the next time the situations occurs in real life. Evaluate the effects of the new response on yourself:

   on others:

Examine Pros and Cons

Although changing to assertiveness can have many benefits, any change can also result in something being taken away. Before you firmly decide on your first assertiveness goal, it is important to examine the pros and cons of acting on an assertiveness goal of your choice. Learning to take a look at the advantages and disadvantages of an assertiveness decision is an important skill. You don't want to rush into an impulsive action and then regret it. Complete Exercise 20, "Trade-offs," now.

EXERCISE 20 Trade-offs

Directions: First name your assertiveness goal, then list the advantages and disadvantages of that goal. Aim to have an equal balance between advantages and disadvantages. You may wish to ask a friend to look at your list and discuss it with you to identify advantages and disadvantages you've missed. Also, try to list the opposite of each advantage in the disadvantage column. For example, increased status (advantage) may lead to decreased free time (disadvantage).

A. **Assertiveness goal:** _____

Advantages	Disadvantages
1.	1.
2.	2.
3.	3.
4.	4.
5.	5.
6.	6.

B. Based on your list of advantages and disadvantages, consider whether the trade-offs are worth the risks involved in being assertive. Write your thoughts here.

C. What advantages would you trade off because of a disadvantage?

D. Cross off one advantage you would be willing to give up because the disadvantage is too great.

E. Now revise your decision in question B, if necessary, based on your crossed-off list.

F. If you find that the disadvantages of attaining that goal outweigh the advantages to you at this time, go on to another goal and repeat the process or use the space below to examine the pros and cons of another of your assertiveness goals.

(continued)

EXERCISE 20 (*continued*)

Assertiveness goal:	
Advantages	**Disadvantages**
1.	1.
2.	2.
3.	3.
4.	4.
5.	5.
6.	6.

You're ready to set your first assertiveness goal. Write it here along with the date you plan to implement it:

Once you've tried out the new behavior, evaluate its effect. Do you feel good about the outcome? Is there anything you'd change? If so, try out the new behavior again, changing it until it feels right. Practice with a role-playing pal or just speak into the mirror in your bathroom or tape record your comments until they sound the way you want them to. Once you're satisfied, you're ready to go on to the next situation in your list of priorities. Continue on, working up to your last (most difficult) situation. By then, you may have new challenging situations.

Use Behavioral Contracts

Behavioral contracts are especially useful in family situations. Successful contracts require changes that include words like "I want"; and consequences, as in "I will take responsibility for." For example, in a family where meeting curfew is a problem, alternative ways to meet curfew could include coming home at a prearranged hour, calling a half hour early to negotiate a curfew that is an hour later, averaging curfew times (e.g., out until midnight one night and in by 8 the next for an average curfew of 10 P.M.), or coming home 1 hour early in exchange for the use of the car.

Successful contract negotiation requires that ideas be clearly stated. For example, if your client says, "I want my husband to be more affectionate," help her translate that general idea into specific behaviors such as, "My husband kisses me good-bye when leaving for work." It is more constructive to focus on contracts that create new behaviors rather than ones that emphasize stopping old behaviors. For example, it is easier to smile than it is to stop frowning; to have one meal together with the family than to stop eating out alone. Behavioral contracts should also include a stated reward following the desired behavior. Here are some examples of contingencies you can teach clients to set up with their family members:

- When homework is finished, Rob can watch TV for 1 hour.
- When clothes are picked up for 3 days in a row, Mary receives a written promise to be taken to a movie, followed up by actually being taken to the movie.
- In exchange for eating one meal a week with the family, Emily does the dishes for David for 2 nights.
- When Mrs. Romero completes her physical therapy exercises, she can sit outside by the garden for an hour.
- When Mr. Davidies finishes the vital signs on all assigned patients, he can go for a 15 minute break.
- When Sarah obtains a card signed by her teacher indicating that school assignments have been completed, she can do whatever she wishes after school that day. Her father will monitor the contract and her mother promises not to nag him, in return her father will be allowed to go out one night a week with his friends.

Go on to Exercise 21 and start writing your own practice situations.

EXERCISE 21 Writing My Own Practice Situation

Directions: Now that you have identified some situations you wish to practice, use the following space to plan a practice situation. Include mirror exercises, audiotape practice, videotape replay, and/or role-playing.

1. The practice situation is:

2. Counterproductive attitudes I hold about this area of assertiveness are:

(continued)

EXERCISE 21 (*continued*)

3. The strategies I will use to practice are:

4. Plans that I have made to try out the behavior in a real-life situation are:

5. I plan to evaluate my progress in this area by:

6. I will reward my accomplishment in this area by:

7. I will write the following behavioral contract for this goal:

CHALLENGING YOUR "SHOULDS"

If you're a woman, part of who you are is based on socialization into being a female. Messages that many women (and some men) commonly receive in our society are that you "should" think of others first, never brag or tell others positive things about yourself, always listen and be understanding, never complain, be attuned to what the other person is thinking and feeling, and be willing to give to others. These messages can make you especially susceptible to guilt induction from authority figures such as supervisors, teachers, or administrators. Even family members can evoke guilt. Some guilt inducing messages are "You *should* work overtime, you're needed," or "You *should* do whatever your boss asks of you because this is part of your work," or "You *should* do whatever your family asks of you, whenever they ask." If you are susceptible to such attempts to make you feel guilty, you probably believe the myths perpetuated through socialization in your family, school situations, and work environment. Examine your own "should" system by completing, Exercise 22, "Challenging My Shoulds."

EXERCISE 22 Challenging My Shoulds

Directions: List the "shoulds" you hold. Many have been with you since childhood, but you may also have developed some during the period of your schooling, employment, or from your spouse or children.

"Shoulds" I hold include:

1.
2.
3.
4.
5.

Go back and look at your list. Now challenge your "shoulds" by explaining why they are counterproductive to your sense of power.

1.
2.
3.
4.
5.

Based on your challenges, decide which of your "shoulds" you will give up and list them, changing them to more assertive statements.

1.
2.
3.
4.
5.

IDENTIFY WHAT'S UNMANAGEABLE IN YOUR LIFE

When your life feels unmanageable, it can sabotage your work, relationships, and life. Several reactions can result in feeling powerless. These reactions include negative control and resentment (Mellody & Miller, 1990). Antidotes include changing yourself by learning assertive "I-messages," letting go and forgiving the other person, changing your self-talk, and practicing relaxation and guided imagery to reduce your anger and stress.

Eliminate Negative Control

Do you live in constant reaction to others around you instead of being proactive? If you do, you probably end up trying to control other people's reality. This is in contrast to positive control that involves actively determining what you will look like, feel, think, and do. Exercise 23 will help you determine if you are using negative control and contributing to the feeling your life is unmanageable.

EXERCISE 23 Assessing Negative Control

Directions: Check yes or no to each of the following questions.

	Yes	No
1. Do you try to control other people so you can feel safe and comfortable?	—	—
2. Do you tell others what they should wear or look like or what action to take?	—	—
3. Do you try to convince others their thinking is wrong?	—	—
4. Do you try to convince others that their feelings are invalid?	—	—
5. Do you let other people control you by telling you what to think, feel, or do?	—	—

If you answered yes to one or more of the questions, you are probably adding to your feelings of powerlessness. The first step in reducing powerlessness is to identify the specific instances of negative control. Write a paragraph about each item you answered yes to.

Practice Positive Control

Empowering yourself to practice positive instead of negative control involves focusing on you, not on the person you're controlling. For each situation you listed in Exercise 11 (page 32), move from thinking, "The problem is the other person," to "This is my problem and I have to solve it." Even if the problem is due to offensive behavior on the other person's part, the most you can do is ask the person to stop. That person may stop or may not. Then you are still back to changing yourself so you can live comfortably with the situation (Mellody & Miller, 1989).

Some ways to do that are as follows:

• Write a letter to your manager, client, or whomever you're angry with, focusing on the reasons for your anger toward that person. Put the letter away and reread it at least a week later. If that doesn't help, make an appointment with a mental health nurse practitioner or psychologist to process your letter in a session.
• Find a colleague to help you role-play the situation, focusing on ways to develop nondefeating strategies for handling angry feelings.
• Attend assertiveness training classes to learn constructive ways to express your feelings and opinions.

Go on to Exercise 24 now.

EXERCISE 24 Moving Toward Positive Control

Directions: Go back and look at the incidents you listed in Exercise 23 and remember specific instances. Ask yourself, what would be a healthier response in each case? (Clue: a healthier response is one that focuses on you and what you can do.) Your answers must include acknowledging your anger and/or uncertainty and on how you can let go of trying to control the other person.

More healthy responses to situation 1:

More healthy responses to situation 2:

More healthy responses to situation 3:

Release Resentment

You feel resentful when you think someone has committed a grievous offense against you. (This is not the kind of resentment you feel because you were mistreated in childhood, which is best dealt with in psychotherapy sessions.) Adult resentment includes obsessing about the incident and reliving the resentment. You can learn self-care measures to deal with this kind of resentment. The anger is strong and you want the other person to be punished because you believe it will reduce your suffering (Mellody & Miller, 1989), but there are ways to deal with it. Go to Exercise 25 and describe incidents about which you have been or are still resentful.

EXERCISE 25 Things I Feel Resentful About

Directions: Fill in the columns below.

Situations that make me feel resentful	What I've done to change the situation

Now go back and look at the situations that make you feel resentful. Think about ways you can change yourself so you don't feel resentful. Some examples of healthier responses follow. Choose the one that seems most reasonable depending on your resentment.

1. Some people's behavior can be hurtful and inexplicable. My best response in such situations it to experience the hurt, accept that it happened and is beyond my control. I will turn the situation over to a higher power and go on with my life. If the person or situation comes back to haunt me, I will say to myself, "I will not let this situation upset me," or "My job is to focus on _____ and I will not get sidetracked."

2. I will have a few sessions with a mental-health nurse practitioner or psychologist and work on releasing my resentment through self-hypnosis, guided imagery, or other cognitive-behavioral approaches.

3. I will use my anger to take care of myself. I will write down a script for what I will say to the person who has ridiculed [demeaned, physically attacked, or exploited] me. I will specifically describe what is happening, for example, "I'm feeling attacked" [demeaned, exploited, etc.]; and what I am feeling such as, "and that hurts [angers, etc.] me." Tell the person what you would like him or her to do differently: "I would appreciate it if you stop attacking [touching, belittling] me."

Realize the person may not change even though you are assertive and speak directly to him or her about the problem. To reduce disappointment, develop a secondary plan, including describing what you can do to reduce contact with this person if he or she doesn't act on your request; "I can't spend time with you anymore," for example. Go to Exercise 26 for ways to do that.

EXERCISE 26 Ending Resentment

Directions: Identify the situations you still feel resentful about and for which the solutions you tried didn't work. Write them down in the left hand column. In the right hand column write down one of the three solutions above and try them out. If that solution doesn't work, go to your second, and if necessary, your third choice.

Situations I'm still resentful about   *Proposed solution*

CONCLUSIONS

Becoming assertive is an ongoing, lifelong task. No one is completely assertive or completely nonassertive. By practicing the principles exhorted in this chapter on a regular basis, you will gradually become more assertive. Have patience and chart your progress.

Remember, you have a right to be assertive and to express your thoughts and feelings.

REFERENCES

McKay, M., Rogers, P. D., & McKay, J. (1995). *When anger hurts: quieting the storm within*. Oakland, CA: New Harbinger.

Mellody, P., & Miller, A. W. (1989). *Breaking free: A recovery workbook for facing co-dependency*. New York: Harper & Row.

Thomas, S. P. (1998). *Transforming nurses' anger and pain: Steps toward healing*. New York: Springer.

3
Calling on Energetic and Holistic Resources

Live your beliefs, and you can turn the world around.
—Henry David Thoreau

If you're not healthy, you can't be empowered. A holistic approach to empowerment includes taking action to rev up your energetic resources, including nutrition, fitness, touch, stress management, and interpersonal support activities. To be fully empowered, you will need to have a healthy body, a calm mind, and adequate support from the people around you. Keep reading and find out how to make sure each of these resources is available to help empower you.

NUTRITIONAL EMPOWERMENT

Are you letting what you eat zap your energy? Certain food substances can deplete you:

- Coffee, tea (caffeinated), cola drinks, and chocolate can aggravate anxiety and panic episodes because too much caffeine can lead to irritability, anxiety, and mood swings.
- Sugar can send your blood sugar on a roller-coaster ride, which can sap your energy and trigger stress symptoms.
- Alcohol is a depressant that can increase fatigue, combativeness, anxiety, and agitation.
- Dairy products can be difficult to digest, thereby worsening depression, fatigue, and anxiety.
- Fruit juice can destabilize blood sugar because it is not the whole fruit and thus can increase fatigue, anxiety, and mood swings.

• Red meat contains saturated fat used to manufacture hormones called prostaglandins that worsen muscle tension, a common symptom of stress.

Take Nutritional Action to Empower You

Specific nutritional actions you can take to empower your body include the following:

1. Drink enough water every day. During your normal daily activities your body loses about 10 cups of water. During exercise, while overheated, and when under stress, even more water is needed. Coffee and cola drinks are not good replacements for water because they contain caffeine, which flushes even more water out of the system. When you experience pain, drink at least a full glass of water. Many kinds of pain are due to dehydration.

2. Eat five or six meals a day if you have low blood sugar. Signs of low blood sugar include sugar craving, depression, fatigue, weakness, palpitations, headache, or feeling jittery. Eating five or six meals at spaced intervals that are high in protein and low in carbohydrates can help balance your insulin production and help you think more clearly and act more assertively.

3. Eat breakfast. Eating a good breakfast will give you a good start for your day and provide your brain with sufficient nutrients to think and talk clearly.

4. To reduce stress, replace depleted nutrients. Stress can deplete you of vitamins and minerals, especially the antioxidant vitamins A, C, and E, the B vitamins, and the minerals calcium and magnesium. You can find all of these in foods. The most commonly lost nutrients are vitamins B and C, commonly called the stress vitamins.

• To replace vitamin B, increase your intake of brown rice, chicken, legumes (dried beans, peas, peanuts), sea food, sunflower seeds, green leafy vegetables, soy products, and sweet potatoes.
• To replace vitamin C, eat strawberries, citrus fruits, broccoli, tangerines, green peppers, honeydew melons, cooked broccoli, cantaloupe, papaya, Brussels sprouts, cooked cauliflower, parsley, onions, tomatoes, and kale.
• Eat plenty of fruits, vegetables, and nuts; they protect you from the internal and external wear and tear of stress. Nuts are also

good energy sources. Some nuts that have been associated with less stress and even less heart disease include almonds, pecans, macadamias, hazelnuts, pistachios, and walnuts.

• Eat foods high in vitamin E, including almonds, wheat germ, olive oil, peanuts, the outer leaves of cabbage, raw spinach, whole-grain rice, asparagus, cornmeal, eggs, sweet potatoes, and leafy portions of broccoli or cauliflower.

• Eat foods high in magnesium and calcium, such as dark greens, tomatoes, broccoli, sardines, almonds, soy milk, tofu, whole grains, fresh peas, brown rice, swiss chard, and figs.

• Eat vegetables or bean soup to ease stress and give you a warm, soothed feeling.

• Have a crunchy snack of popcorn, raw vegetables, rice cakes, or a fresh apple to relieve stress by using vigorous chewing.

5. To keep you on an even keel, eat complex carbohydrates. Have a baked potato, a plate of pasta, or some rice and vegetables to calm you down. Complex carbohydrates raise your level of serotonin to naturally tranquilize you. Complex carbohydrates can lift your mood and help you resist eating high-fat and high-sugar foods. Having a handful of grapes or a slice of whole-wheat bread or a bowl of bran cereal can help give you the steadiness and lift in mood to help you take action to empower yourself. Some especially high-satisfaction foods include potatoes, fish, oatmeal, oranges, apples, whole-wheat pasta, baked beans, grapes, whole-grain bread, popcorn, bran cereal, eggs, cheese, white rice, lentils, brown rice, and rice crackers.

6. Reduce stress by eating foods high in fiber. High-fiber foods can give you a feeling of fullness, short-circuiting the urge to binge, gain weight, and, as a result, feel depressed. Eat more digestible fibers including whole-grain breakfast cereals, fruit, vegetables, dried beans, whole-grain breads, nuts, and seeds. Steer clear of high-fiber foods that are sugary or contain sugars. They deplete you of energy (after the initial high) and make you want more. Feeling energetic is halfway to feeling empowered.

7. Reach for magnesium, not chocolate. Do you crave chocolate? This substance is often used as a self-medication for dietary deficiencies, especially magnesium (Bruinsma & Taren, 1999). Chocolate is high in sugar and nonuseful fat. Both are disempowering. Instead of reaching for the chocolate, try eating food high in magnesium. Eat a slice of whole-grain bread, a bowl of cereal with wheat germ, a handful of nuts, a couple of figs, an orange or tangerine, soy milk, fresh peas, brown rice, Swiss chard, or a salad of green leafy vegetables.

8. Eat foods high in B vitamins to reduce stress. If stress and anxiety are keeping you from feeling empowered, the B vitamins can enhance your mood and calm you. A recent review of the research on the effect of nutrients on mood reported four double-blind studies that concluded an improvement in just one of the B vitamins, thiamine, was associated with improved mood (Klipstein-Grobusch et al., 1999).

Use Ayurvedic Principles

Ayurveda means "daily living knowledge." It is both a system of health and healing and a philosophy of life. It had its origins on the Indian subcontinent 3,000 to 5,000 years ago. Ayurveda is an integration of mind, body, and spirit and fits into a holistic paradigm. There are five basic elements: earth, air, fire, water, and space. These five elements come together and give rise to the energy, *dosha,* or force that regulates the body. Three doshas or body types occur: *vata, pitta,* and *kapha.* Specific foods calm and nurture each mind/body type. Identify which type you are by reading the descriptions below (Collinge, 1996; Lonsdorf, Butler & Brown, 1993).

Vata: If you're a vata, you tend to be active, alert, and restless. You must be involved in activity to feel well. You have a lot of energy, but you may not direct it appropriately. You disperse and sometimes waste energy and money. You'd probably rather be a musician or artist than an employee of someone else. Too much vata gives you butterflies in the stomach, fear, worry, insomnia, vertigo and emptiness, and a general feeling of not being grounded. It can also manifest as dryness (of the skin, nails, colon, bowels, nose), osteoarthritis, or osteoporosis. If you're a vata type, you may wake up energetic, but be tired by afternoon. You're probably very funny and charming.

To keep balanced and empowered, favor warm, cooked foods and avoid cold foods and drinks and large amounts of salads and raw vegetables so your mind will be clear and your energy directed appropriately.

Pitta: If you're a pitta type, you transform energy, taking one thing and turning it into something else. When you're feeling balanced and healthy, you're decisive, efficient, passionate, and hungry for life. You have a sharp mind and you're intense, sometimes with a sharp tongue, but would make a great CEO because you "budget" and transform energy into effective projects. You probably have a fiery personality, a lot of anger, irritability, a red face, aggressiveness and competitiveness, stress-associated heart conditions, ulcers, colitis, skin disorders, early graying, and excessive hot flashes. Avoid hot spices, tomatoes, vinegar, alcohol, refined sugar, and other acidic or pungent foods to keep yourself balanced and calm.

Kapha: If you're kapha, you're heavier, slower moving, calm, more solid, and have great muscular strength. You may be tranquil, steady, stable, and grounded. You accumulate money and energy and may bury your head in the sand or become a couch potato. When you're feeling healthy, you are unflappable, loyal, a genuine comfort, and a great middle manager. When you're stressed, it may manifest as sinus problems, asthma, diabetes, chest colds, and retention of water. Your personality can get congested, too, when you're stressed and you might drag your feet, become complacent, heavy-hearted, and greedy. Eat a diet rich in vegetables, fruits, and legumes (peanuts, dried beans), and lighter on sweets, meat, dairy products, and fatty foods in order to feel stable and grounded.

Many people are a combination of two types. Foods to eat that pacify both pitta and vata types are shown in Table 3.1.

Complete Exercise 27 now to set goals for adding nutritional solutions to your empowerment agenda.

EXERCISE 27 Setting Nutritional Goals

Directions: Choose at least two of the nutritional solutions described above and write a specific goal for each.

Use the following format. For best results, share your goal with a trusted other and ask to receive a gentle query and reminder weekly to help you meet your nutrition goal.

I, _____ [your name], agree to eat at least two servings of_____ [foods] a week.

I, _____ [your name], agree to eat the following foods to balance my Ayurvedic type:

TABLE 3.1 Pacifying Foods for Pitta and Vata Types

Animal products:	Eat chicken or white meat of turkey primarily. Egg whites are okay and so is a small amount of shrimp; venison is all right. Avoid beef, egg yolk, lamb, pork, seafood, and rabbit.
Vegetables:	Eat mostly sweet and bitter vegetables, cucumber, green beans, zucchini, parsnips, and okra. Also eat moderate quantities of leafy greens, lettuce, parsley, and sprouts with olive oil dressing (no lemon or vinegar).
Fruits:	Eat sweet fruits (dark grapes, mango, sweet oranges, sweet pineapples, sweet plums, prunes, figs), avocado, coconut.
Legumes:	Eat only mung beans and tofu.
Grains:	Eat cooked oats, basmati rice, white rice, and wheat.
Nuts/seeds:	Coconut, sunflower and pumpkin seeds.
Condiments:	Coriander, cardamom, fennel, turmeric, cinnamon, and a little black pepper.
Sweeteners:	Avoid molasses, white sugar, and honey.
Dairy products:	Unsalted butter, milk, cottage cheese, and ghee are okay.
Oils:	Olive, soy, sunflower, and coconut.

PHYSICAL FITNESS

Physical exercise is an important solution to the problem of feeling stressed, depressed, and disempowered. A large study of 3,402 participants found that men and women who exercised two or three times a week experienced significantly less depression, anger, cynical distrust, and stress than those who exercised less frequently (Hassmen, Koivula, & Uutela, 2000). According to a review of physical activity and mental well-being published in *Public Health Nutrition,* there are now several hundred studies and more than 30 narrative or meta-analytic reviews of the potential for exercise to reduce subclinical depression and anxiety, improve self-esteem and mood state, and enhance resilience to stress.

The exercise you engage in need not be aerobic or intense for you to enhance your feelings of well-being and reduce stress. One study showed that swimming or yoga can enhance mood and energize (Berger & Owen, 1992). You don't have to do anything strenuous to achieve benefits. Even nonstrenuous, leisure physical activity can provide a buffer against the physical signs of stress and anxiety due to feeling disempowered (Carmack, Boudreaus, Amaral-Melendez, Brantley, & de Moor, 1999).

Choose a fitness activity that works for you. Exercise 27 provides information about the best exercise to reduce stress and anxiety, increase self-esteem, and sleep better. If you choose weight lifting, martial arts, or any more strenuous activity, make sure you either enlist the assistance of a trainer or read extensively so you will exercise safely. There are three rules to follow no matter what the activity is:

1. Build up to your level of exercise gradually.
2. Listen to your body. Stop if you feel any pain, light-headedness, or fatigue.
3. Pay attention to the weather or room conditions and dress so you will be sufficiently warm or cool.

Complete Exercise 28 now.

EXERCISE 28 Exercise That Empowers

Directions: Check off the exercise that suits you best, then write two goals using the format you select.

___ dance, martial arts, or weight lifting* to increase your self-esteem
___ walk, bike, dance, or practice martial arts to sleep better
___ ballroom or line dance, garden, or walk to enhance joy and feel relaxed

I, _____ [your name], agree to _____ [exercise activity] for at least _____ minutes at least 5 times a week starting _____ [date].

I, _____ [your name], agree to _____ [exercise activity] for at least _____ minutes at least twice a week starting _____ [date].

*If you have high blood pressure, avoid weight lifting.

Have trouble getting yourself to exercise? It may be because you are giving yourself excuses for not exercising. Here are some tips for disputing each excuse.

1. I'll exercise tomorrow. Now is the time I've set aside to exercise, so it's important to do it now. This will give me a feeling of empowerment, while making an excuse can disempower you.

2. I'm already worn out. Exercise will energize and empower me, so now is the time to exercise. My fatigue is mental fatigue and a good physical workout is what I need to balance my body, mind, and spirit.

3. I'm too busy to exercise. There is nothing more important than me and my health. I will keep exercise a high priority. It takes time to exercise, but I'm worth it!

4. I don't feel well. Unless I have a fever or a stay-in-bed sickness, exercise is good for me. I will take it a little easier than usual, but I will go out and exercise. It will make me feel better even if I only exercise for a few minutes.

5. I'm not motivated to exercise. I can get motivated by reminding myself that I just have to start exercising and I'll start to feel the results; it will get easier and easier as I go.

6. I'd rather watch TV in my spare time. Watching TV is a waste of time. If I'm committed to empowering myself, I will turn off the TV and start exercising.

7. Other things take precedence over exercising. Only because I let them. Taking care of myself is as important as anything else. I'll be able to do other things more efficiently, I'll be healthier, and I can even put my mind on cruise control and think about these other things while I'm exercising.

8. I didn't get enough sleep last night. I can rest later. For now, exercise is important and research has shown that exercise leads to better sleep. Meanwhile, exercise will energize me.

9. It's not a big deal if I miss my exercise session once in a while. It is a big deal. I promised myself I'd exercise and my commitment to me is the most important commitment I can make.

If you still need more motivation for exercising, examine Table 3.2 for tips on starting and sticking with your exercise program.

TOUCH

Touch is a powerful tool for growth and healing. Research has shown that just holding someone else's wrist can slow the person's heartbeat and reduce blood pressure, and gently touching the shoulders can have measurable physiological effects such as reduction in heart rate (Richards, McMillin, Main & Nelson, 2001). A daily back rub can reduce anxiety levels in children and adolescents (Feltman, 1989) and adults (Simington & Laing, 1993; foot

TABLE 3.2 Tips for Starting and Sticking with Your Exercise Program

- Start small. Don't think you can jog 2 miles your first time out. Walk half a block instead. Caution is always best. If you're significantly overweight and over 30 years old, check with your health care provider before you start exercising.
- Wait for 2 hours after a meal to exercise.
- Wear brightly colored clothes and reflectors when exercising outdoors at night.
- When running, walking, or skiing, search out smooth surfaces for safer exercise that protects your joints and feet.
- Use proper equipment and clothing.
- Have fun. Pretend you're an Olympic race-walker and put a banner across your chest. Do whatever you have to do to make your exercise session fun and joyful.
- Walk after every meal, even if it's only for 5 minutes. It will mark a definite end to eating and jump start your metabolism.
- Treat your exercise sessions like any other important activity: Block out the half hour or hour on your calendar and let nothing interrupt you.
- Focus on the time you spend exercising, not on what you accomplish. You'll be more consistent if you just put in the time, especially when you don't feel up to par. Then, when you feel great, go all out.
- Work exercise into your daily routine by parking a few blocks away from your destination, walking upstairs instead of taking the elevator, walking or dancing at lunchtime or on your break, mowing your own lawn, carrying your own groceries, etc.
- To reduce boredom vary the type of exercise. Use weights one day, walk the next, swim the next or take a Tai Chi class. No matter what you do, include at least 10 minutes of warm-up and cool-down stretches to avoid injury.
- Use imagery to encourage yourself. Picture yourself eager to exercise or picture yourself toned, radiant, energetic, and healthy after your exercise session.
- Focus on the positives of exercising. Keep a record of your moods, energy, relaxation, concentration, bowel habits, and sleep patterns and correlate it with your exercise patterns.
- Work with a supportive peer or trainer or join an exercise club if you have difficulty motivating yourself. Being around people who value exercise will rub off on you. Spend less time with couch potatoes and naysayers who derogate exercise. If they harass you, ask them to either join you or leave you alone.

acupressure and massage can decrease pulse and respirations and increase quiet time (Sutherland, Reakes, & Bridges, 1999); therapeutic touch can reduce anxiety (Gagne & Toye, 1994), massage can increase health status (Mathai, Fernandez, Mondkar, & Kanbur, 2001) and sedate (Smallwood, Brown, Coulter, Irvine,& Copland, 2001); acupressure can reduce nausea (Norheim, Pedersen, Fonnebo, & Berge, 2001); and skin-to-skin contact between mothers and their infants in intensive care can enhance healing in the babies and provide self-esteem, mastery, and meaning to the mothers (Affonso, Bosque, Wahlberg, & Brady, 1993).

Interestingly, touching someone when you don't feel well can affect them negatively (Wirth, Richardson, Martinez, Eidelman, & Lopez, 1996). Even your plants can benefit from touch according to James Cahill of the University of Alberta. The simple act of touching them can have a dramatic effect on whether they thrive because it can cause them to release chemicals that affect their growth and ability to fight off insects, the researchers speculated. If that's the case with plants, touching another human probably confers healing qualities, too.

Human beings need touch to stay healthy and well. There are many ways you can meet this need. One way is to collect many daily hugs from a family member or friend. Another is to give back rubs and foot rubs to your partner and family members and receive similar treatment from them. You could also obtain a massage from a massage therapist. There are many books available that teach the novice how to massage another person or use acupressure. Many nurses practice and teach therapeutic touch, including how to provided therapeutic touch for yourself and your family. Reiki is another touch therapy you might find useful. Please explore these possibilities and make sure you obtain sufficient positive touch every day. Not only will it empower you, it can enhance your mood and immune system. When all else fails, give yourself a massage. Directions appear in Table 3.3.

TRAIN YOUR STRESS RESPONSE

As mentioned in chapter 1, feelings of stress and anxiety often lead to disempowerment.

TABLE 3.3 Directions for Self-Massage

Step 1: Sit in a quiet place where you won't be disturbed. Rub your hands together until they feel tingly.

Step 2: Use your fingers and hands to convey a loving touch and continue to breathe deeply and easily throughout the rest of the steps.

Step 3: Gently massage your head and scalp. Massage the back of your head to the base of your skull, spending extra time on any sore or tight spots. Massage the top, side, and back of your ears.

Step 4: Caress and massage your forehead. Massage your checks lightly. Use three fingers of both hands to gently massage the bony areas around your eyes, nose, and chin.

Step 4: Stroke firmly up your throat to your chin. Use a circular massage motion with your fingertips all around the back of your neck. Move your head from side to side, probing with your fingers for sore spots. Spend extra time on those and experiment with pressure, tapping and stroking across the muscle.

Step 5: Use your right hand to knead and massage your left shoulder and down your left arm. Knead your left thumb, each of your fingers on your left hand, and the palm and top of your left hand.

Step 6: Use your left hand to knead and massage your right shoulder and down your right arm. Knead your right thumb, each one of the fingers on your right hand, and the palm and top of your right hand.

Step 7: Use your left or right hand to massage your chest and abdomen.

Step 8: Use both your hands to massage as much of your back and buttocks as possible.

Step 9: Move your hands to the upper part of your left thigh. Use both hands to massage down your leg. Massage your feet, massaging each toe, top and bottom, between the toes, and the sole, heel, and sides of your feet. Observe how your left leg and foot feel compared to your right leg and foot.

Step 10: Repeat the massage process with your right thigh, leg and foot.

Step 11: Observe the effect on your whole body. If there are any parts of you that desire more massage, tend to them gently and lovingly.

Optional step: Either before or after your massage, use a loofah sponge on your bare skin to bring healing energy and blood to your back, legs, and arms.

Training your stress response can be helpful. The first step is taking control. Sometimes it may not seem as if you are in control of yourself or your behavior, but you are. Let's take a look at some common life situations and see who's really in control. Go to Exercise 29 now.

EXERCISE 29 You Are In Control!

Directions: For each of the following behaviors, check whether you or someone else is in control.

Behaviors	You're in control	Somebody else is in control
When you eat	_____	_____
What you eat	_____	_____
Brushing your teeth	_____	_____
Combing your hair	_____	_____
Going to bed	_____	_____
Traveling to work, school, or to shop	_____	_____
Drinking	_____	_____
Smoking	_____	_____
Taking drugs	_____	_____
Exercising	_____	_____
Reading the newspaper or a book	_____	_____
Paying your bills	_____	_____
Deciding what to say	_____	_____

See, you do control many things in your life. Take a deep breath and enjoy that feeling of empowerment. Granted, other people do influence you to some degree, but you have control over your daily activities—some of the most important things you can do to stay well and enjoy life. To reduce stress and anxiety, faithfully practice the skills described in the next exercises.

When you're upset, you probably breathe in the upper part of your chest. Anger, fear, anxiety, tension, shame, and other negative feelings can take over your breathing patterns unless you've trained yourself to deep breathe before these feelings arise. Go to Exercise 30 and practice it now and whenever you need to relax.

EXERCISE 30 Learn to Deep Breathe

Directions: For best results, record the following directions into a cassette and play them back when you're ready to practice deep breathing. Be sure to read the directions in your most calm and peaceful voice. Pause when indicated by dots for at least a few seconds.

1. Find a quiet and peaceful spot . . . someplace where you feel relaxed and alone . . . Put a Do Not Disturb sign on your door . . .
2. Kick off your shoes and loosen any tight or restrictive clothing . . .
3. Lie or sit down in a comfortable spot . . .
4. Place one hand on your abdomen . . .
5. Close your eyes and gently suggest to your abdomen to push your hand out as you breathe in . . .
6. Exhale, feeling your abdomen retract . . .
7. When you're ready, inhale again, keeping your hand on your abdomen . . .
8. Keep breathing in and out in a relaxed manner . . . letting your hand move in and out with your abdomen . . . experience more and more feelings of calm with each breath.

Meditation can also help you reduce stress. There are many different kinds of meditation. The kind you're going to be using includes saying one statement as you breathe in and another statement as you breathe out. Alternative statements are also provided. Go to Exercise 31 now and complete the meditation. Practice it daily. Awakening and prior to sleep are suggested.

EXERCISE 31 Stress-Reduction Meditation

Directions: Follow the steps below. If you wish, record them into a cassette using a calm, slow voice.

1. Breathe in and say to yourself, "I am relaxed and calm . . ."
2. Breathe out and say to yourself, "I let go of whatever it's time to let go of . . ."
3. Continue breathing in and out, repeating the two phrases.

Alternative statements:
"Peace."
"Forgiveness."

Besides using deep breathing and meditation to reduce stress and empower yourself, you can also use structured relaxation. Go to Exercise 32 now and practice structured relaxation.

EXERCISE 32 Structured Relaxation

Directions: Read the following directions into a tape recorder and play them back often. The more often you listen to the tape, the easier it will become for you to feel relaxed. If you find the tape relaxing, at the least play it upon awakening and at bedtime. You can play it in the background at other times, but not while driving or using other equipment.

Pause after each sentence and use a calm, monotone voice. Find a quiet, private, and peaceful spot. Kick off your shoes and loosen any restrictive clothing. Lie or sit down in a comfortable place.

1. Close your eyes and focus your attention on the tape and the words you hear . . .
2. Let your breathing move easily and slowly to your center . . .
3. Think about how slow and relaxed your breathing is getting . . .
4. Experience the sensations of your body relaxing . . .
5. If any thoughts come to mind, let them drift away . . .
6. If the thoughts persist, set them aside with a mental note to return them when you finish this exercise or at whatever time is best for you . . .
7. Focus your attention on your left foot . . . Notice how heavy and relaxed it is becoming . . .
8. The next time you inhale, send a wave of relaxation to your left foot . . .
9. The next time you inhale, send a wave of relaxation up your left food and all the way up your left leg . . . let it flow up your left hip . . . let that wave of relaxation flow up your left side to your shoulder . . . up your neck . . . up your head . . . and let it flow out the top of your head . . .
10. Now focus your attention on your right foot . . . the next time you inhale, send a wave of relaxation to your right foot . . . and all the way up your right leg . . . let it flow up your right hip . . . let that wave of relaxation flow up your right side to your shoulder . . . up your neck . . . up your head . . . and let it flow out the top of your head . . .
11. The next time you inhale, send a wave of relaxation to your right foot and up your right leg . . .
12. The next time you inhale, send a wave of relaxation up both your feet . . . up both your legs . . . let that relaxation move up your body . . . up your hips . . . up your abdominal area . . . up your chest and back . . . up your neck . . . through your entire head . . . letting it flow out the top of your head . . .
13. The next time you inhale, scan your body for any areas that need relaxation . . . the next time you inhale, send a wave of relaxation to those areas . . .

(continued)

EXERCISE 32 (*continued*)

14. Keep breathing and letting waves of relaxation flow through you . . . enjoy the positive sensations of relaxation . . . feeling more and more calm and empowered . . .

Another kind of stress reduction procedure are the positive statements called *affirmations*. They are based on the theory that thought patterns create experience. This metaphysical causation explanation insists that by changing thinking patterns, experience can be changed (Hay, 2000).

How often do you make comments such as, "That's the way things are. They'll never change."? What you are really saying is that *you* believe things will never change. A belief is just an opinion, something you've incorporated into your belief system of how the world operates, something you look for incidents that verify your theory. Holding this belief, you are apt to overlook or discount incidents that don't fit in with your belief system.

On the other hand, if you begin to say, "Things are changing all the time. I can be part of a positive change," or "I am empowered," you will be more apt to observe and look for incidents that support that theory. Hay (2000) says that if you find yourself saying a statement more than 3 times, write it down. It has become an affirmation. While you're learning to put more positive thoughts in your statements, you may hear yourself still repeating negative affirmations. When you hear one, merely say, "Cancel that," and continue on with your life. Go to Exercise 33 now, Reducing Stress with Affirmations, and follow the directions.

Exercise 33: Reducing Stress with Affirmations

Directions:

1. Say one or more of the following affirmations at least 20 times a day.
2. Write at least one of the affirmations below on 3 x 5 cards and place them in prominent places where you will see and read them frequently.

I am calm and peaceful.
I have the strength, power, and will to empower me and those around me.
I trust all life processes: I am free and empowered.
Everything that happens is empowering.
With every breath, I am becoming more and more empowered.

Tips for Easing Stress

Here are some tips for easing stress on the job or off:

- Get up a few minutes earlier so you don't feel rushed.
- Get enough sleep. It's best to go to bed and wake up the same time every day to keep balanced and rested.
- Take the pressure off yourself and give yourself permission to be imperfect.
- When stressed, take a few deep breaths and try some stretching exercises.
- Pay attention to the messages you're giving yourself and say STOP to negative thoughts and CANCEL if you've already had the thought.
- Focus on your accomplishments when you feel frustrated and pat yourself on the back. You're wonderful!
- Set realistic expectations. Consider what's reasonable to accomplish in the time period you have.
- Encourage patients, clients and caregivers to participate in their own care. It will take the pressure off you and contribute to them becoming whole persons.
- Celebrate your wholeness by paying tribute to aspects of you that aren't job-related. Furnish your locker or deck with items that comfort you and remind you of supportive family or friends.
- Tune into your spiritual and emotional side while you're working. Fill your needs related to them throughout your work day. Maybe say a prayer to help you achieve your goals, or tune into your life purpose by seeing today in perspective as the small picture, not the big picture. Release strong feelings by picturing them floating away as a color or comic strip character
- Take care of your intellectual side by checking a book out of the library on your break or on the way back from a meeting. Meet your social needs by sharing one thing about yourself with one person each day.
- Instead of thinking it's the end of your world when you fail, look at the flip side and name at least one thing that's positive about the way things turned out.
- Make sure your schedule reflects your priorities.
- Each day complete a "must do" list and make sure you accomplish them before you leave. Be sure to congratulate yourself for completing your list.

- Avoid self-medicating. It only masks the underlying source of your stress. The ability to handle stress is within you.

REFERENCES

Affonso, D., Bosque, E., Wahlberg, V., & Brady, J. P. (1993). Reconciliation and healing for mothers through skin-to-skin contact provided in an American tertiary level intensive care nursery. *Neonatal Network 12*(3), 25–32.

Berger, B. G., & Owen, D. R. (1992). Mood alteration with yoga and swimming: Aerobic exercise may not be necessary. *Perceptual Motor Skills, 75,* 1331–1343.

Bruinsma, K., & Taren, D. L. (1999). Chocolate: Food or drug? *Journal of the American Dietetic Association, 99,* 1249–1256.

Carmack, C. L., Boudreaus, E., Amaral-Melendez, M., Brantley, P.J., & de Moor, C.(1999). Aerobic fitness and leisure physical activity as moderators of stress-illness relation. *Annals of Behavioral Medicine, 21,* 251–257.

Collinge, W. (1996). *The American Holistic Health Association complete guide to alternative medicine.* New York: Warner.

Feltman, J. (1989). *Hands-on healing.* Emmaus, PA: Rodale Press.

Fox, K. R. (1999). The influence of physical activity on mental well-being. *Public Health Nutrition, 2*(3A), 411–418.

Gagne, D., & Toye, R. C. (1994). The effects of therapeutic touch and relaxation therapy in reducing anxiety. *Archives of Psychiatric Nursing, 8,* 184–189,

Hassmen, P., Koivula, N., & Uutela A. (2000). Physical exercise and psychological well-being: a population study in Finland. *Preventive Medicine, 30*(1), 17–25.

Hay, L. (2000). *Heal your body: The mental causes of physical illness and the metaphysical way to overcome them.* Carlsbad CA: Hay House.

Klipstein-Grobusch, K., Grobbee, D. E., den Breeijen, J. H., Boeing, H., Jofman, A., & Witteman, J. C. (1999). Dietary iron and risk of myocardial infarction in the Rotterdam Study. *American Journal of Epidemiology, 149,* 412–418.

Lonsdorf, N., Butler, V., & Brown, M. (1993). *A woman's best medicine: Health, happiness, and long life through Ayur-veda.* New York: Jeremy Tarcher/Putnam.

Mathai, S., Fernandez, A., Mondkar, J., & Kanbur, W. (2001). Effects of tactile-kinesthetic stimulation in preterms: a controlled trial. *Indian Pediatrics, 38,* 1091–1098.

Norheim, A. J., Pedersen, E. J., Fonnebo, V., & Berge, L. (2001). Acupressure against morning sickness. *Tidsskr Nor Laegeforen, 121,* 2712–2715.

Richards, D. G., McMillin, D. L., Mein, E. A., & Nelson, C. D. (2001). Osteopathic regulation of physiology. *American Academy of Osteopathy Journal, 11*(3), 34–38.

Simington, J. A., & Laing, G. P. (1993). Effects of therapeutic touch on anxiety in the institutionalized elderly. *Clinical Nursing Research, 2,* 438–450.

Smallwood, J., Brown, R., Coulter, F., Irvine, E., & Copland, C. (2001). Aromatherapy and behaviour disturbances in dementia: a randomized controlled trial. *International Journal of Geriatric Psychiatry, 16,* 1010–1013.

Sutherland, J. A., Reakes, J., & Bridges, C. (1999). Foot acupressure and massage for patients with Alzheimer's disease and related dementias. *Image: Journal of Nursing Scholarship, 31,* 347–348.

Wirth, D. P., Richardson, J. T., Martinez, R. D., Eidelman, W. S., & Lopez, M. E. (1996). Non-contact therapeutic touch intervention and full-thickness cutaneous wounds, a replication. *Complementary Therapies in Medicine, 4,* 237–240.

4

Saying Yes to Your Needs and No to Impossible Demands

When there is no enemy within, the enemies outside can't hurt you.
—African proverb

Why is it so hard to say yes to our needs and dreams? Probably because from babyhood we've been taught to be nice, to do what our parents say, and to conform. This may have worked when we were helpless infants, but adults must be able to take care of themselves and to cooperate and collaborate with others. Assertiveness is one way to do that.

Assertiveness involves saying what you mean and meaning what you say. If you're not clear stating what you need or don't want, there is very little chance others will oblige. Take a look at Table 4.1 and see why the statements in first column aren't likely to achieve the response you want, while the statements in the second column are.

Before you attempt to be assertive, you have to grapple with the risks of doing so. Do you imagine all sorts of dire consequences for acting assertively? You may have been brought up in a household where you were taught to hold your tongue, to be quiet and sit down. These assumptions about what might happen if you're assertive need to be examined in the clear light of day. Let's take a look at some of these counterproductive beliefs.

1. If I'm assertive, I might upset the other person. This is a common fear. The fact is, some people may not like it when you are assertive, but you have every right to express your feelings. Avoiding the situation can only lead to a buildup of anger, a blowup, and then guilt. It could even lead to serious interpersonal problems that could take a tremendous emotional toll (which is often converted into physical symptoms) on all involved. Remember,

TABLE 4.1 Saying Yes to Your Needs—Assertively

Nonassertive comments	Assertive comments
You don't appreciate me.	I'd like a written evaluation of my work.
You should have called.	If you're going to be late, please call so we can reschedule.
You didn't hear a word I said.	Please listen to my opinions, even if you don't agree with them. I want to talk to you about some things that are bothering me. I want to talk to you about our discussion yesterday. For me it isn't finished.
We never discuss anything.	Let's sit down and talk together with no interruptions.
I never get a chance to have input in decisions.	I want a say in decisions that affect me. I'm starting to feel resentful and I don't want to feel that way so please let me choose what we do every other time.

if you approach people with respect, showing sensitivity to their feelings and being honest about yours, the chances of upsetting them are greatly lessened. Be sure you avoid belittling or putting others down. Even then, an upset could occur, but it will probably be short-lived and could lead to resolving a more upsetting situation. You will have to decide if you want to take a risk and be assertive. If you don't speak out, the situation may never be resolved. Even if the other person reacts badly, you were able to express yourself. Feel good about that. You will also learn firsthand what the other person is about. You will know what you're up against. By remaining silent, you'll never know.

2. If I'm assertive, the other person might try to get back at me. There is no guarantee that the other person won't get back at you no matter what you do. You goal is to be assertive, not control the other person's reactions. It would be nice if every time you were assertive the other person said, "I understand what you want and I'm going to change right now." Most of the time that won't happen. Being assertive means you respect the other person's right to be assertive, aggressive, or avoiding. Pick your fights. You may not wish to be assertive with a boss or teacher or anyone who holds the power to affect important outcomes for you. Think situations through and decide if the risk is worth the potential result.

3. If I'm assertive, I might fail and look silly. It's true that the other person may not do what you want. You're not failing if you're being assertive. You are being an important role model for the other person and anyone who observes you. Even if the other person doesn't go along with your assertive request, you still have options. You can always say, "I'm sorry you feel that way. This issue is very important to me. I hope you'll think about it and decide to talk to me about it at another time." Even if the other person makes fun of you, discourages your attempts, or calls you overly emotional, you still have options. Take what the person says and incorporate it into your attempt to convince, for example, "That's right, I am emotional about this and I'm going to keep talking to you about this until we resolve it." This lets the other person know that you cannot be pushed around and does it in a mature and well-thought-out way.

BEING ASSERTIVE RESPECTS THE OTHER PERSON

Some people think assertiveness is rude. There is no reason for assertiveness to be disrespectful. You can be polite and still be assertive. When you're assertive, you describe the facts without embellishing or manipulating. You express how you feel without blaming the other person, for example, "I feel upset about being teased" or "I get angry when I'm not listened to." Once you've expressed your feelings, you can then ask for action in a polite way, such as, "Please finish your report as we agreed" or "Please acknowledge my contribution to the effort." To add an extra quotient of respect, restate the other person's viewpoint or feelings while maintaining your position: "I hear that you're angry, but this is important to me" or "I understand this isn't important to you, but I feel better when we finish on time."

By respecting and verbalizing the other person's feelings or viewpoint, there is no need for defensiveness or attack. The stage is set for clear communication and a win-win situation. There has been no attempt to strip the other person of dignity or violate that person's rights. You have remained respectful, but clear in your communication.

LEARNING TO DISAGREE AND STILL GET ALONG

One dynamic that occurs in families, especially dysfunctional ones, is the inability to allow disagreement. Everyone must agree, or at least pretend to, to reinforce the myth of a close family. The reality is that if you get two people together for any length of time, they will disagree. That is because we are unique individuals with unique thoughts, reactions, and dreams. Although the idea may be scary to you if you've been raised in a dysfunctional family, learning to disagree and still get along is a high priority skill in assertiveness.

Why do so many people go to almost any extreme not to disagree? Again, it's no doubt a learned behavior. We may have been threatened or forced to comply, often with words of dire consequences if we do not. Old messages die hard.

Let's take a look at how assertive disagreeing differs from aggressive disagreeing. Assertive disagreeing includes statements such as, "I heard what you're saying, but I disagree" or "I understand your viewpoint, but I'd like you to listen to mine." You will notice that an assertive disagreement always respects the other person's point of view, but lets the other person know that you have a different opinion or viewpoint.

Aggressive disagreeing can run the gamut from disrespecting the other person to verbal threats or physical attack. No matter what form it takes, it never respects the other person's point of view. There is no attempt to come to a compromise or to collaborate. There is only an attempt to force the other person to comply. This can also take a passive-aggressive form. In this case, the other person can act too weak, too fatigued, or too helpless, thus forcing you to comply, often by caring for him or her instead of assisting in a growth process.

RESOLVING CONFLICT

Conflict can keep you from attaining your goals if you are using a lot of energy to resolve it. Conflict includes many behaviors, from quiet arguing, to quarreling, to outright physical aggression. Conflict happens in all relationships, but if it's excessive or if you are physically harmed by someone, it's time to find a counselor or talk to the police.

Conflict can be healthy. If there isn't any, it could mean that one of the people in the relationship is too submissive or may be stockpiling hurts. Take a moment and think about whether there is positive conflict in your relationships or if you are submissive or have stockpiled resentment. Conflict can be stress-producing, so you will no doubt want to resolve it unless it is the kind of conflict that is promoting open communication. If you ignore conflict it's apt to go underground, but it will still affect you and can surface at unexpected times.

You can get into conflict if you assume that other people see things the way you do. Often, it just isn't true. You may hate confrontations and be a very private, laid-back, trusting, warm, quiet, sympathetic person who prefers to listen. When you do show your feelings, others may tell you to stop being overly emotional, which may make you feel victimized and cause you to shut out the other person so you stay in control.

You may think everyone else is like you are. Many people don't decide things based on feelings. They're more concerned with facts and although they want to control things, too, they may be animated, decisive, enthusiastic, manipulative, and confrontational. It you appeal to their feelings to solve a conflict, you'll get nowhere. They'll want the last word and may change the topic to put themselves in a good light; and although they're confrontational, if you confront them, they may strike back hard.

Some people analyze everything and are serious, sensible, methodical, and self-controlled. They may pride themselves on being emotionally uninvolved. If you confront them about their lack of feeling, they may hit back hard, too, attacking any weakness in your reasoning, losing patience, trying to regain control, or getting depressed.

Other people have great charm and style and appear to be somewhat aloof and removed from feeling, but they try to establish a superior position in relation to you. They rarely display extremes of behavior or high emotion. They won't raise their voices or disagree violently, but they may often look depressed or self-absorbed. When you call them on their behavior, they may cut you off, become even more depressed, boil over with anger.

Which one of these descriptions is you? Which one describes your family members, boss, peers, and friends?

Think about it for a while. It's important to know your style and which communication style is used by the other important people in your life. Once you figure that out, you can start to resolve any conflicts you have with them because you can anticipate what they will do and need and provide it. For example, it would be crucial to speak to the "analyzer" by using logical reasoning and keeping your feelings to yourself. With the "fact finder," present just the facts, and be sure to provide plenty of praise for the "charmer."

Also read nonverbal communication. This may take some practice, but you have probably been reading and responding to nonverbal communication for years. You may just need to think more about it to bring it to the forefront of your mind. Bringing this information into conscious awareness will provide you with even more clues about how to reduce conflict. When what is said conflicts with facial and body movement, pay attention to gestures. They are probably the most clear communication indicator in those circumstances.

The face is probably the easiest part of the body to read because the muscles of the face react to stress and are easily seen. Keep in mind the person's "normal" look. Also watch for eyebrow, forehead, lip and tongue changes. Watch for tics or spasms when feeling is running high. Be aware of changes in skin tone. Reddening or paling can communicate a mood shift. The eyes can betray emotions that are not being shared in words. Train yourself to read them.

Once you know what's behind a conflict situation, there are other ways to plan for a resolution. One way to do this is to be willing to listen actively to each other and to address underlying issues. Good negotiation skills are necessary in this process. All relationships provide a study in negotiation. To get along with another person, you must be willing to give and take. Many people never learned these skills. If you don't, consider taking an assertiveness course.

Claiming is an important part of conflict resolution. Claiming includes verbally owning your feelings when you are upset. Here are some claiming statements: "I feel angry when I'm teased" or "I take full responsibility for the message."

Blaming messages communicate that the other person in the relationship is responsible for your feelings. For example, "You make me so angry when you tease me." The "you" word is usually a clue that blame is about to be attributed. If you accuse the other person, there is a good chance you will hear a defensive or blaming comment in return. You can turn blaming statements into jointly owned issues with comments such as, "As a family, we don't talk honestly with one another," or "Our family doesn't show much affection and I wish we did," or "As a department, we don't inform each other of important issues."

Quarrels are not a good conflict resolution tactic. During quarrels, one person's values are attacked. Insults and personal attacks are often hurled in the heat of a quarrel. The result can be many bad feelings. To prevent quarrels, try to do the following:

- Identify the times when quarrels are most apt to occur and avoid discussions at those times.
- Note what triggers quarrels for you and use stress management procedures to reduce them.
- Identify the danger signals that led up to the conflict and refuse to engage in another quarrel.
- Agree on a "no fight" signal when everyone involved is in a neutral emotional state. A communication time-out (making a T with your two index fingers) can be used or any other signal that is agreed upon prior to a quarrel. If the sign alone doesn't stop bickering, say, "Time out. We'll talk later," and leave the area until you've cooled down. It will also help to defuse conflict if you reinforce the other person's self-image.

Communication experts D. G. Foster and M. Marshall (1994) suggest some ways to get through to important people in your life.

- To people who focus mostly on feelings, you might say (using as much warmth as you can muster), "I like that you're always so thoughtful and try hard not to hurt other people's feelings. You never try to dominate or make a decision without carefully considering every aspect of the situation, and for that I'm grateful."
- To people who are self-controlled, you can say, "I like that you're always so coolheaded in a crisis, that you always fight for what you believe in, that you're systematic and focused, and that you can make sense out of the most difficult information."
- To people who are really hardworking, you could say whole-heartedly, "I like that you get so passionate and enthusiastic about everything, that you always deal with things quickly and efficiently, that you're such a hard worker, and that you're never a follower, always a leader."
- To people who try to be superior, you can say in a respectful tone, "I like that you're so exciting to be around, that you really make things happen, that you get to the heart of everything, and that you have so much charisma."

Once the important people in your life have a sense of being understood by you, it will be easier to talk with them and resolve any conflicts that arise. Go to Exercise 34 now and apply what you've learned about conflict resolution.

EXERCISE 34 Resolving Conflict

Directions: Identify a past conflict situation and use the information about conflict resolution to plan a way to circumvent conflict in the future.

1. Describe a recent conflict situation in which you were involved. Include the outcome.

2. Consider the information above about conflict resolution and identify the characteristics of the people involved: are they hard workers, charmers, feelers, self-controlled, superior acting or something else?

3. Devise a specific plan for preventing conflict with the person(s) involved in the conflict.

SAYING NO AND STILL GETTING ALONG

Why is it so hard to say no to others? Probably because we've learned from our childhood to say yes to our parents and teachers. Rocking the boat can bring about resistance because people just don't want to have to deal with unexpected situations. It's so much easier for some to use intimidation to force others to go along with their goals.

The problem with this method is that it results in employees and family members who feel angry, depressed, apathetic, dissatisfied, burned out, and even physically ill. By becoming more assertive, you can limit the chances of having these negative feelings. Having a say and being rewarded for creative ideas and actions are important to most workers.

Allowing yourself to become run-down by demands to help others, to work unreasonable hours, undertake unreasonable or unsafe tasks, and doing nonjob-related tasks are examples of an inability to say no. If you are very tired, frustrated, or hungry, you cannot be providing a high-level performance for your boss or your loved ones.

Another reason it's important to say no is that it can help you to avoid becoming involved in situations you think you may regret later on. Saying no can often allow you to keep your respect, and it decreases the chances that you will feel exploited, abused, taken advantage of, or manipulated into doing something that you do not choose to do. When you feel this way, resentment is bound to build up. Resentment is counterproductive to health and to the attainment of your work goals. Saying no allows you to direct your life by making decisions, keeps you from getting sidetracked onto irrelevant tasks or issues, and allows open communication. Saying yes when you mean no is dishonest and indirect communication.

Whenever you are asked to grant a request, resist the impulse to blurt out the first answer that occurs to you. First, be sure you understand the request. If you do not understand it, ask for clarification until you do. Often clients and coworkers will make a request that seems simple and straightforward. On exploration, it may turn out that more or something different is being requested than you first thought. If you hear a vague, innocent-sounding request, be on the alert and decide to explore the request further. Remember that some people in your work environment may seek to capitalize on your fear of appearing ignorant if you ask for clarification. If you allow this fear to win out, you may end up making decisions that are not based on sound judgment.

Be aware that you have the right to postpone making a decision unless an emergency or life-threatening situation is involved. It is both appropriate and desirable to postpone many decisions. In some situations it is particularly important to postpone decision making, such as when a major career change is involved, when you do not have all the information you need, and when you see advantages and disadvantages to granting the request and are unable to decide logically which decision is best. Try not to make premature decisions just because someone is pressuring you to do so. Also, it is important to avoid justifying or explaining your decision once you have said no. When a no sounds apologetic or unsure, the other person will know that you are wavering and may continue to pressure or badger you. On the other hand, once you have given a response, further requests by the other person may begin to seem pushy, inappropriate, and inconsistent with your rights in the situation. If others continue to badger you after you have given a definitive answer, you can ignore the request or repeat your previous answer until you have been heard. Resist the impulse to answer questions about why you said no, unless you feel comfortable doing so. Refuse to get sidetracked by answering insults or insinuations.

There are many reasons why it's important to say no when your work conflicts with your emotional, physical or spiritual health. You're the expert on when this conflict may occur. Your boss will just roll along, thinking everything's okay; or maybe, in the worst-case scenario, forcing you to go along by using threats or other nonholistic methods.

If you are licensed personnel and your boss requires you to work below your licensure, you're accountable for your own actions. Your license is the legal process that authorizes you to perform designated skills and services. You owe a greater duty and are more accountable to your clients than to your boss. According to Gloria Ramsey, RN, JD (2002a), "employers cannot require you to work below your licensure." To be sure, check your employee handbook and your state's practice act. Read them both and know the grounds for disciplinary action, penalties for dishonorable conduct, and your obligation to uphold your practice act and see that others do so as well. When your employer subjects you to liability and there is an incident, you'll be held accountable. The best way to say no to acts that put your practice in jeopardy is to state: "This is a violation of my practice act, my employment agreement, and standards of practice." State your objections clearly and specifically, follow up in writing, and make a copy for your records, including a statement of who you are and what your qualifications are. If you do accept an assignment that violates your practice act, you are responsible for that assignment, and if you leave you could be charged, so say no before accepting.

The same holds true if you're given an assignment and you aren't prepared to fulfill it. If you're asked to supervise other personnel and you're a licensed person, there may be legal and ethical implications of undertaking this assignment. Say no, in this case or ask for a refresher course and time to hone your skills (Ramsey, 2002b).

Choose your situations well. You don't want to go around saying no to every demand your boss makes of you. It's just not realistic. But there are situations when it will important for you to refuse, and you'll probably need practice in doing so since most of society has been taught to say yes. See Exercise 35 for examples that can help you learn to say no effectively.

EXERCISE 35 Saying No

Directions: This exercise will give you varied practice in saying no. Try each example.

1. Practice saying the word no until you sound convincing and confident. When you think you can say no in a convincing manner, find a friend or coworker and ask for feedback about how you sound. If necessary, ask for suggestions for how to sound more convincing.

2. Practice saying the following comments aloud until you and your partner agree you sound firm and confident. Take them one at a time, mastering each one and then moving on to the next.
   a. No, I don't understand that. Please explain what you mean.
   b. No, I can't decide now. I need some time to think it over. How about if we discuss my decision on Thursday?
   c. No, I can't help you with that now. I'll help you in half an hour.
   d. No, I can't do that report now. I'm doing something else now.
   e. No, I can't give you the full report now, but I will give you the first part.
   f. No, I can't work overtime today.
   g. No, I cannot accept an administrative position.
   h. No, I won't change my mind, and I'd appreciate not being asked again.

3. List some work or home situations in which you need practice saying no.
   a.

   b.

   c.

   d.

   e.

   f.

4. Choose one or two of these situations and rehearse your response with a partner. Make sure you say the word no, at least once. If necessary, devise a role-playing situation or behavior rehearsal situation to use as a basis for your practice.

EXERCISE 35 (continued)

5. Try out your rehearsal response in the real-life work or home situation and evaluate the results. If necessary, discuss the results and practice again with your partner.

Because it is often so difficult to say no you may need additional practice. If this is a priority goal for you, don't hesitate to do whatever is necessary to enhance your skills by continuing to role-play and evaluate your performance. For more ideas about saying no, see Exercise 36.

EXERCISE 36 Designing "No" Comments

Directions: Three situations are provided for you to practice designing what you might say to refuse a request. REMEMBER: You do not need to make up an excuse or apologize. Also, avoid preaching to your friend. Be sure to stick to the issue of covering for your friend. Once you have filled in assertive responses, practice saying your lines with a partner. A model response for this situation follows:

Situation 1

A friend of yours wants you to cover for him at work. This is a habitual situation and you've decided to take a stand.

Friend: Say, would you mind covering for me? I have to leave early.
You: _____

Friend: Come on, just this once.
You: _____

Friend: I don't see why you won't help me out.
You: _____

Friend: Boy, you're some friend.
You: _____

Friend: All right, I'll get someone else.

Model Response

Friend: Say, would you mind covering for me? I have to leave early.
You: No, Sam. I can't cover for you.
Friend: Come on, just this once.
You: I'd like to, but I can't cover for you.
Friend: I don't see why you won't help me out.

(continued)

EXERCISE 36 (*continued*)

You:	I just can't cover for you.
Friend:	Boy, you're no friend of mine.
You:	I am your friend, but I can't cover for you.
Friend:	All right, I'll get someone else.

Situation 2:

Your boss has asked you to take a leadership position. You have considered the offer carefully and have decided you cannot accept it at this time. You are about to say no.

Boss: Well, what is your decision?
You: _____

_____

Boss: What? Pass up an opportunity of a lifetime? This may never
come up again.
You: _____

_____

Boss: You have the skills and ability for the job. You have to take it!
You: _____

_____

Boss: It is your duty to take this position.
You: _____

_____

Boss: Well then, whom do you suggest for the position?

You may wish to record the above situations and then listen to your responses, shaping what you say until you are pleased with your words. Once you have perfected what you want to say, try your comments out in real-life situations.

Saying no to impossible demands includes saying yes to your needs. It also includes dispelling counterproductive beliefs.

DISPELLING COUNTERPRODUCTIVE BELIEFS

Counterproductive beliefs are beliefs you hold that keep you from feeling empowered. Some commonly held counterproductive beliefs include the following:

- I am responsible for other people's feelings.
- I should always be understanding and caring.
- I should never make a mistake.
- I should be able to handle whatever workload I am assigned.

- I should live with what is, since I can't change it.
- I should never tell anyone about my special skills, since that would be bragging.
- I should never say no to a request for help.
- I should never take a risk because it might prove fatal.
- No request is too unreasonable.
- I can't say no to a boss because the boss always knows best.
- If I was really good at my job, I'd be able to do whatever is asked of me.
- It my boss asks me to work late or do extra tasks, I should do it, otherwise I'll be viewed as uncooperative.
- It's easier to grant a request than to face what will happen if I don't.

It is imperative that you identify these and other counterproductive beliefs that can keep you from reaching your goal of assertiveness. Remember that the consequences of most interactions are neutral, or at least less important than we often assume. Even if they do have consequences, you need to decide how important it is for your health and self-esteem to speak up and be heard. Some questions you might use to begin the process of challenging your counterproductive believe appear in Exercise 37.

EXERCISE 37 Challenging Your Counterproductive Beliefs

Directions: Choose one of the counterproductive beliefs you hold. Write down your answers to the following questions to help you challenge counterproductive beliefs that may be keeping you from feeling empowered.

Counterproductive beliefs I hold:

1. Is this belief so?

2. Why do I think it is?

3. What evidence do I have that the belief is true?

(continued)

EXERCISE 37 (*continued*)

4. Does this belief help me to feel the way I want to feel?

5. Does holding this belief help me achieve my goals without hurting others?

6. Does this belief help me to achieve my goals without hurting my physical, emotional, social, or spiritual health?

7. Does this belief deny my rights as a person?

8. Does my belief decrease significant short- and long-term unpleasantness for me?

9. If I were the other person in the interchange, would I be devastated by an act of assertiveness?

10. Does this belief seem overprotective of myself or others?

11. Could one assertive act really result in the negative consequences I expect?

12. How would I feel if I were in the other person's position?

13. How would I feel if I were in the other person's position?

In order to answer question 13, you need to be able to evaluate your ability to be assertive. (If you're unable to answer this question as the other person in a situation, find a friend who will role-play the situation to identify how others might feel if you're assertive.)

EVALUATING YOUR ABILITY TO BE ASSERTIVE

Part of saying no is the ability to be assertive in the way you present yourself to others. There may be cultural or situation variables that necessitate an adaptation of the evaluation criteria. In those cases, modify them or look for assertive role models in your environment and imitate their behavior. At first, it is helpful to focus on only one or two evaluation criteria. Avoid trying to be totally assertive in all areas at first practice or real-life situation. As you gain skill, focus on one or two other criteria. Not all criteria will be pertinent for all situations, so choose those that seem most relevant and focus on them. For example, if you are talking on the telephone, eye contact, facial expression, gestures, body posture, and positioning are not important. Likewise, some evaluation criteria related to active work orientation, and constructive work habits may not be applicable to assertive interchanges with clients or consumers. Part of your evaluation is your satisfaction with your performance. If you are not satisfied with it, you are not apt to make that behavior part of your future repertoire. When evaluating your performance, consider whether you were pleased with all or part of your performance and whether you choose to continue to work on that aspect at this time.

Even if you initially choose to focus on a particular aspect of assertiveness, it doesn't mean you cannot change your mind and your goal. At the same time, it is important not to give up too easily. Whatever you choose to do, continue with the current focus or switch to another, and be sure to reward yourself either for your performance or for taking the responsibility to set your own goals or choosing to change them. Reward yourself by thinking, saying, or writing a word of encouragement or praise to yourself. Or reward yourself by doing one of your favorite activities. Once you begin to feel more comfortable with your new assertive behavior, simply engaging in it will make you feel empowered and rewarded. The Assertive Evaluation Criteria appear in Figure 4.1.

Steps to take when developing assertive behavior are:

1. Assess yourself in the skill area.
2. Appraise the interpersonal and work situation to determine your rights and responsibilities and to identify short- and long-term behavior consequences.
3. Decide the ideal behavior for that situation.

FIGURE 4.1 Assertive evaluation criteria.

Presentation of Self
Initiated conversation
Used clear, concise statements
Stayed focused on the issue
Expressed thoughts and opinions openly
Shared feelings
Used "I" or "we" statements
Spoke in a clear, firm, fluent voice
Maintained eye contact
Used appropriate facial expression
Used gestures that enhance what was said
Used open body posture
Sat or stood at appropriate distance

Active Work Orientation
Suggested a change
Worked to full capacity
Told others my expectations
Clarified what others expect from me
Set short- and long-term goals
Worked to achieve short- and long-term goals
Let others know of my special work skills
Set and held to deadlines and time limitations

Constructive Work Habits
Limited interruptions
Concentrated on one task
Planned to complete unpleasant tasks
Said no to illegitimate requests
Structured work day for satisfaction, reward, or empowerment

Giving and Taking Criticism, Evaluation, Help
Accepted a compliment
Gave a compliment
Owned up to a mistake or limitation
Pointed up a mistake or limitation in a neutral way
Asked for assistance
Remained calm while being observed or evaluated

Control of Anxiety or Fear
Felt comfortable while:
Standing up for my rights
Disagreeing
Expressing anger
Dealing with another's anger
Handling a put-down or teasing
Asking for a legitimate limit to workload
Taking a reasonable risk

FIGURE 4.1 (*continued*)

Satisfaction with Performance
Liked my performance
Liked parts of my performance
Did not like my performance, but plan to try again
Did not like my performance, and choose not to work on this goal
Rewarded myself for my assertive performance or choice

---

4. Plan and practice the desired behavior in a safe, comfortable environment.
5. Try out the desired behavior in a simple, real-life work situation.
6. Identify and dispel counterproductive beliefs that may prevent you from being assertive.
7. Evaluate your behavior using the Assertive Evaluation Criteria.
8. Reward yourself for your assertiveness.

ASSERTIVENESS STRATEGIES

There are many strategies you can use to improve your presentation of self. These include mirror practice, audiotape practice, videotape replay, observation of assertive role models, development of a peer support and role-playing network, and design of your own assertive exercises.

Mirror Practice

Observe your posture, gestures, and facial expression in a mirror. It can give you feedback or information about how you present yourself. Practicing an assertive speech while looking in a mirror can help you be sure that your words and actions present an integrated message as well as give you practice in maintaining eye contact. Once you get over the self-consciousness about talking to a mirror, you can benefit greatly from this kind of practice. It is especially useful when you do not have a trusted peer with whom to practice.

Find a quiet spot for practice, a place where you will not be interrupted. If necessary, hang a Do Not Disturb sign on a bedroom or bathroom door before practicing. You can use a large mirror to focus on total presentation of yourself, or a smaller mirror to focus on your facial expression. Get to know how you look to yourself when sitting with legs crossed and open, when standing with your arms crossed or at your sides, and when expressing thoughts and feelings. A nonproductive belief that you may have about using a mirror is that it is a sign of vanity. On the contrary, it is important to get to know yourself before deciding what assertive actions you choose to take. Finding out how other people might see you is an important aspect of getting to know who you are. Use the mirror exercise, Exercise 38 now.

EXERCISE 38 Get to Know Yourself

Directions: Use a small mirror for this exercise. It works best if you ask someone else to read the directions aloud. Be sure to take sufficient time to do each part and reflect on its meaning.

Step 1. Look into your eyes in the mirror. Make eye contact for at least 30 seconds. Time the eye contact to make sure that you have a sense of how long 30 seconds is. At the end of 30 seconds, reflect on or discuss your reactions. For example, what did you feel, see, and think while making eye contact with yourself?

Step 2. Now look at the rest of your face closely. What do you see? Describe your face aloud, being sure to assess physical traits, feelings, or expressions you notice. What do you like about your face? Reflect on or discuss what you felt, saw, or thought while looking at the rest of your face.

Step 3. Close your eyes and visualize a pleasant situation or spot, a place where you are relaxed and comfortable, someplace where you can go to feel good. Concentrate until you have that picture clearly in your mind. Now open your eyes and look at your face. Does it look relaxed? Do you feel comfortable? If not, how could you use this exercise to learn to relax your face? Reflect on or discuss how the degree of relaxation or tension shown in your face may affect your assertiveness.

Step 4. Now take a few minutes to reflect on or discuss your reactions to this exercise.

Audiotape Practice

Tape recorders can provide helpful cues to you about how you sound: whether you sound like you want to sound, or pause too frequently; whether you speak too softly, loudly, or quickly; whether your voice conveys the feeling you hope to communicate; and whether you stick to the issue. It is not unusual for people not to listen to what they say or how they say it, and tape recorders present an accurate account of what was said. Although the inexpensive ones may distort your voice quality somewhat, the words you say, pauses, and other valuable information will be reproduced. If you have never listened to yourself on tape, do not miss this experience. At first, you may feel self-conscious and be disappointed in what you hear. In time, you can learn to be a more critical listener and change those aspects of your speech that you are not satisfied with. One way to experiment with your voice on audiotape is to read a poem in which you raise and lower your voice and pitch. This will give you a feeling for how you can vary and control your voice. Though many women speak in a high-pitched voice (especially when anxious or uncomfortable), a firm, lower-pitched voice sounds more assertive.

Too many pitch variations are apt to sound as if you are over-emotional or even out of control, but no pitch variation can be boring. You may tend to increase the rate of speech when you are anxious or angry, but if you practice with the tape recorder, you can learn to tell yourself to slow down. You can also practice stressing important words, which will also result in a more assertive presentation. Another idea is to record your part of all phone conversations for several days. (Do not attempt to record the other person's conversation because that is illegal unless you have their consent.) Be sure to mention the other person's name near the beginning of the conversation. You may wish to keep a notebook or pad near the telephone to record the time, date, topics, or general theme of the conversation and your perception of how you felt and sounded. Do not listen to the tape for 3 days. At the end of that time, listen to the tape from beginning to end and try to correlate it with your written notes. This exercise will help you to learn more about how you sound when feeling different ways, when you hesitate, and what special speech patterns you use.

You can also use the tape recorder to provide instant feedback. For example, you may wish to say a sentence and then play it back to hear how it sounds. If you like the sound, move on to the next word, phrase, or sentence you wish to work on. If you didn't like the sound, simply rerecord it, or if you wish, erase what you said and record again. This kind of exercise is especially useful when you have difficulty saying certain words (such as no) or phrases (I'm angry). The following are words and statements you could use for practice in this manner:

- I cannot talk to you now.
- I'm angry.
- I don't want to discuss it now.
- I disagree.
- I made a mistake.
- I appreciate your help.
- I like your work.
- No.
- I'm upset about the way things are.
- I want to talk with you about this.

Videotape Practice

Videotape feedback is an important tool in learning assertive behavior. Participants have reported that viewing themselves on a videotape monitor was the most significant learning experience they had during a 2-day assertiveness training workshop.

Some elements of presentation of self that can be studied and modified through videotape and replay of the taped segment are eye contact, body posture and positioning, gestures, facial expression, latency of response, brevity of assertive statements, and adequacy of delivery. Videotape provides the truest representation of how you present yourself to others.

Despite its benefits, many participants have initially been resistant to being videotaped. Because equipment is involved, it is wise to enlist the assistance of a technician (when holding a workshop) or (if you're doing this on your own) a friend who is well-versed in operating the camera and replay equipment. Many small things can lead to a delay in replaying a videotaped segment, especially if your assistant is not an expert. The initial apprehension of participants can also be a deterrent. Nevertheless, once you see the benefits that can accrue in a brief period of time from a videotape learning experience, you will probably want to use it often.

One way to use videotape effectively is to prepare or purchase a short two-person interchange, using assertive role models to depict situations. Any of the role-playing situations in this book could be adapted and used to develop a demonstration videotape. Modeling or demonstration has been shown to provide excellent transfer or learning.

The interchange can be stopped at any point for discussion, and it can be replayed as many times as necessary to study assertive aspects. Most videotape recorders have pause buttons that can be used to freeze the tape while you look at or discuss what is happening at that moment. Pausing to examine what was just said and its effect on the other person's speech and body language is a useful learning experience.

Facial expressions, body positions, and gestures that enhance or detract from your presentation of self are clearly visible. Also, seeing and hearing yourself immediately after you speak can have a great impact on your future behavior. Once you know what to look for in your performance, you can view and critique your behavior without assistance from an instructor. It is usually helpful to view the tape with the person with whom you role-played the segment. That person can help you notice and reflect on your performance. Until you become very skilled and knowledgeable with this medium, it is suggested that you do view (or at least discuss) your videotape performance with another person who possesses assertive skills, preferably a workshop leader.

One of the major advantages of videotape is that it can give you the freedom to experiment with real-life situations, yet it can be erased and redone until your performance pleases you. Using the videotape in a workshop situation away from your work or home situation can also provide safe practice without the possibility of being glimpsed or heard by your boss or peers. If all the employees at your setting participate in a workshop, some of this safety is reduced. Managers can still be placed in separate rooms for practice and then come together near the end of the workshop to practice what they have learned by using real-life situations, with the instructor present to facilitate discussion and follow-through.

This medium offers a way to integrate assertive skill practice in a brief period of time. Real-life skill practice would take much longer because the opportunity for useful practice is not always available, and adequate feedback about your performance may also be lacking. Two- to 3-day workshops have been found effective, at least in the short term for learning basic assertive skills. To keep assertive skills functional, it is suggested that after returning from a workshop, you find a peer support group and continue to discuss and role-play challenging situations. Another suggestion is to schedule regular assertiveness update workshops and then bring in an assertiveness videotape expert to run the sessions.

The video segment can also be used as a standard with which to compare your assertive behavior. Table 4.2 gives points to remember when viewing a videotape or when role-playing a structured, two-person interchange.

Observation of Assertive Role Models

Locate people in your work or social environment who you think demonstrate the assertive behaviors you wish to learn. Spend time with them. If possible, enlist their support in helping you to become more assertive. Praise them for their assertive behavior, and let them know you would like their support and assistance in becoming more assertive. If you feel uncomfortable asking for help, you can increase the time you spend with them. You can learn to become more assertive by being in the company of assertive people.

It is easier to be assertive with people who are assertive. Once you are motivated and know the performance level you are striving for, you will see people who are actively demonstrating the very skills you wish to emulate. Read books and periodicals and choose movies that present an assertive (not a passive, passive-aggressive, or aggressive) approach. Turn off television programs or leave movies that show people as helpless victims, aggressive uncaring individuals, or nonassertive and passive. If you attend a workshop on assertiveness, observe how the leader models skills in assertiveness.

Try to emulate behaviors you observe and like. To assist in this process, begin to set assertiveness goals. Write one or more down on a 3 x 5 card and carry it with you. Read it often. This will encourage you to make assertiveness part of your everyday life. Some goals you may choose include "I am able to state the purpose of an interchange with another person," or "I am able to breathe deeply and stay calm when observed by other people."

Role-Playing and Behavioral Rehearsal

Role-playing is a way of playing a role you hold or wish to hold in real life. During the process, you say and do things you foresee yourself doing and saying or things you have said and done in the past, with a goal of bettering your performance. You can also use *role reversal.* In this situation, you take the role of that person in the scene, generally for the purpose of empathizing with or understanding the perspective of the other person. The more specific you can be about your goal for the conversation and how the other person can make it more vivid or real-lifelike for you, the more apt you will be to transfer what you've learned to the actual situation.

TABLE 4.2 Assertive Presentation of Self in Planned Meetings

1. Set up an appointment well in advance, if possible. "Prime" the other person for the purpose of the upcoming interview or meeting by sending a memo stating the objective of the interview clearly. If you wish, talk to the person and clearly state the purpose of the interview. Of the two actions, the written memo is preferable because it stands as a reminder and permanent record of the purpose and of your initiation of the meeting.

2. Role-play upcoming anxiety-provoking situations with a friend or colleague. Anticipate intimidating or unclear comments and practice responding to them before the actual meeting or interview. *Note:* Every situation has both short- and long-term ramifications, so plan accordingly. For example, although you hope to settle a small misunderstanding with a boss, friend, or family member (short-term goal), you probably also want to leave the door open for cooperation and collaboration in the future (long-term goal).

3. Write down important points or statements on a 3 x 5 card and bring it with you to the meeting. If necessary, read them to the other person, saying something like, "I've written this down because it's very important and I don't want to forget anything." This is preferable to stumbling or forgetting to stay on the topic.

4. At the appointment time, structure the discussion environment for clear and open communication. For example, move chairs to face one another, use direct eye contact, and ask for no interruptions. (You might want to suggest this in your memo, thus allowing the other person to take care of potential interruptions prior to your meeting.) Do not be put off by others' attempts to hurry you or to stray from the proposed topic of discussion.

5. Restate the purpose of the meeting; for example, "I'm here to clarify . . . or, "I want to talk with you about . . . or, "I'd like us to work together to solve the problem . . ."

6. Avoid getting sidetracked onto irrelevant issues. Keep the discussion on the identified issue with such comments as, "Before you go on, I'd like to clarify . . ." or "I'd like to finish discussing . . ."

7. If the other person's tone of voice, facial expression, or nervous movements intimidate you, **concentrate on the words being said.**

8. Use relaxation exercises and deep-breathing techniques to remain calm. Write a reminder to "breathe in your abdomen," or "picture peace and serenity" on your 3 x 5 card. Another idea is to have notepads printed up with a relaxing scene on them and bring that to the meeting with your notes and calming techniques written on one of the sheets.

9. Determine what motivates the other person and use that information to support your argument or purpose. For example, if the other person seems threatened by your comments, reduce the threat by stating that you do not wish to argue or fight, but that you do wish to express

(continued)

TABLE 4.2 (*continued*)

your viewpoint. If the other person is motivated by budgetary concerns, use that to support your argument, for example, "Not only will this program assist employees to be more effective, but it will also save the company money because participants will have learned to be more efficient in their communication and everyday business practices."

10. Keep time limitations well in mind and move the meeting along. If necessary, make comments such as, "We have 10 minutes left and I'd like to come to an agreement on . . . ," Or, "If I don't hear from you about this by Thursday, I'll call you."

Role-playing is a technique that is especially helpful in learning to make assertive response, and it can be used in your peer support group. The process will help you think through your goals, specify problematic situations, sharpen listening and presentation of self skills, and reduce anxiety about being assertive. If you have had negative experiences with role-playing or if you feel there is an unreal or artificial quality to the technique, you may be resistant to trying it. Remember the advantages of role-playing: It offers you a vehicle for safe practice in assertiveness. Try it. With practice, you'll learn to like it and to profit from its use. Merely reading a book or attending a lecture on assertiveness will not lead to behavior change. You will need to actually say the words and examine the effect in order to benefit. Exercise 39 provides some role playing situations to get you started.

EXERCISE 39 Role-Playing Practice Situations

Directions: Study how the situations are presented and the kind of information that is given. You may wish to use the situations as they are or modify them to fit your needs. When writing your own situations, be sure that the written description clearly requires appropriate assertive (not aggressive or avoiding) behavior and that there are at least several statements to which replies can be made. Find a partner who agrees to help you. Be sure this person makes the situation as difficult as possible. Provide coaching so this occurs, for example, "Sound angrier," or "Really try to make me feel guilty." Use one or more of the following situations or use your own real-life situations, but be sure to model them after the information presented here. Rehearse each situation several times or until you feel comfortable with your new behavior. If you like, rewrite the responses of the other person. Evaluate your performance using the Assertive Evaluation Criteria (Figure 4.1)

(continued)

EXERCISE 39 (*continued*)

   1. Saying no. Your boss suggests that you take on added administrative duties, even though others have more seniority than you. You thank your boss for recognizing your ability, but say no, you cannot accept the position at this time. Give your boss several good reasons why you cannot accept. Write in comments by your boss that could make you feel guilty or flattered. Make sure your responses remain a firm no.

   2. Facilitating group work. You are working with a team, but there is no designated leader, or the designated leader is not facilitating the group. Make comments to help the group clarify what they expect from one another, such as, "Let's go around the group and say what we expect from one another." Also ask the group to identify subtasks, e.g., "Let's break this down into small tasks, by making a list of the sub-tasks. I'll start by identifying some of them." Finally, ask the group how they wish to proceed with the subtasks, for instance, "We've got the subtasks identified. How do you wish to proceed?" Make sure to have at least one other person who makes comments such as, "Oh, we already tried that" and "That will never work."

   3. Saying no and setting limits. One of your supervisees keeps requesting extensions on deadlines for writing reports and expects to be excused from assignments the other supervisees meet. Your job is to work this out with the supervisee in an assertive manner. Some suggested comments include "I can't continue to give you extensions on getting your reports done. All my other supervisees are getting their work in on time. We need to work out a way to help you get your assignments in on time. What do you suggest?" Make sure the supervisee presents some excuses for why the work hasn't been done, such as, "I've had a lot of illness and my kid is in jail and my husband just left me. Can't you understand? I just need a little extension."

   4. Dealing with interruptions. You serve on a committee. One of the other members of the committee interrupts your statements before you can finish a sentence. Deal with the situation in an assertive way. Some suggested comments include "Excuse me, but I haven't finished," or "Let me finish my sentence and then you may talk." Make sure the person who is role-playing with you interrupts you at least three times.

   5. Standing up for a promotion. You wish to be promoted, but your boss seems unaware of your talents, downplays your good points, and tries to make you feel guilty that you aren't doing more. You decide to keep a log of the things you have accomplished in your work. After developing quite a few entries in your log, you set up an appointment with your boss to share your accomplishments. Begin the scene as if you have just entered your boss' office. Some suggested comments include "The reason I wanted to meet with you is . . . ," and "I've been keeping a log of my accomplishments and I'd like to share them with you." Make sure the person who plays your boss takes a phone call while you're meeting, rushes out into the hall at least once on a so-called emergency,

(continued)

EXERCISE 39 (*continued*)

and takes out files and records and starts to work on them. Include some statements for yourself such as "Maybe this is a bad time. Let me make an appointment when you won't be interrupted," or "Perhaps we could go to lunch and discuss this?"

6. Dealing with manipulation. You have just left a meeting during which you were able to speak up and give you opinion. No one supported your comment and even ignored what you said, even though you did speak clearly and loudly. After the meeting, one of the group members approaches you in the hall says, "Are you all right? You seemed so upset. You embarrassed the boss by putting her on the spot." Suggested comments include "I'm fine. I didn't intend to embarrass the boss. I was only voicing my opinion." Remember: You have a right to speak up and be heard. Make sure the other person playing the role is condescending, motherly, and overprotective.

7. Disagreeing by asking for a reasonable workload. Your boss changes your assignment without telling you why. You are angry and upset and decide to make an appointment to discuss the matter. During the meeting you would also like to work out a more equitable work assignment. Avoid falling into the trap of feeling guilty. Stick to the point: "Let's get back to discussing a reasonable workload for me." Collaborate: "Can we collaborate on this and find a better way to help me complete this assignment." (Always have some ideas in mind, such as, getting an assist from another employee, rotating the assignment of difficult and demanding tasks, asking if your boss can go to his or her boss to get another person assigned to help with the work.) Be sure to have the boss make some comments like "All clients are your responsibility," and "If our clients need you, you must take on the job."

8. Dealing with others' anger. You enter a workroom and find a peer yelling and screaming at a client. You convey confidence by asking your peer to come for coffee or a cup of tea so you can find out what the problem is and work out a solution. (Always get angry employees out of the triggering situation). Be sure to include some angry comments in the other person's role-playing speeches as well as some resistance to leaving the room with you.

9. Dealing with others' anger at you. A peer meets you in the hall and accuses you of not meeting your responsibilities. Make sure the person who plays the accuser is angry and belittling, for example, "Who do you think you are? Do you think you're better than we are? You aren't doing anything around here to help." Acknowledge the anger ("I hear your anger," or "You sound really angry.") and find out what the anger is about ("What's happening that you're so angry? Give me specifics"). Neither avoid the anger (by looking away, smoothing things over, or changing the subject), nor attack back by sounding angry or accusatory.

10. Telling others about your anger. You have been stewing about a derogatory comment someone made about you in front of others. You decide to have lunch with the person and bring up the incident so you

(*continued*)

can stop stewing. Be sure to include some comments such as "I feel angry about what you said," and "I want to work this out so I'll feel better and we can have a better relationship. I don't want to stay angry at you." Make sure the other role-player tries to avoid a discussion ("I'm too busy to talk about this"), denies making the remark ("I never said that"), and tries to smooth it over ("Come on, don't be angry") without letting the anger be expressed.

A special instance of role playing is *behavior rehearsal.* In this case, you can prepare for upcoming situations by specifying the exact words and situations you think you will have to deal with, and you practice saying and doing the exact things you will have to perform in the real-life situation. You write out a script of exactly what you'll say and exactly what the other person will say. You might want to start out with a script because it is more structured than role-playing. Once you master the role playing process, you can begin to develop your own situations for practice. The script in Table 4.3 presents a behavioral rehearsal situation.

Peer Support

Seek out peers who are working to become more assertive. Ask them to meet with you regularly to role-play problematic situations, to work toward specified assertiveness goals, and to give one another praise and rewards for accomplishing assertiveness goals. Developing a support network or group that disintegrates into complaining about "the system" or how employees are kept down will not be a constructive force for change or learning. If neces-

TABLE 4.3 Behavioral Rehearsal Example

Assertive problem: Sticking to the point.

You:	I want to talk to you about . . . [topic]
Other:	How nice to see you. How have you been?
You:	I've been fine. About . . . [topic] I think we should. . . (suggested solution).
Other:	Say, while you're here, what do you think about the new boss?
You:	Maybe we can talk about that later. Right now, I would like to finish discussing . . . [topic].

sary, put up a notice on the bulletin board in your work area suggesting that others interested in the topic contact you. If possible, convince several of your peers to attend an assertiveness workshop with you. After the workshop, implement the skills and ideas you learned by holding regular peer-group meetings and skill practice sessions. Share ideas about the areas you and the others wish to work on, tell them what comments are helpful to you, and ask them to practice these with you to help you change your behavior. If you have attended a workshop, you probably have learned some helpful comments. If not, the following statements can be used or adapted to your specific situation:

- "Look me in the eyes when you talk."
- "Relax your hands; place them on the chair armrests."
- "Speak more loudly."
- "Say that more concisely."
- "Speak slowly."
- "Emphasize the important words."
- "Turn your body toward me."
- "Tell me the specific purpose of our meeting."
- "Say something to keep our discussion on track."
- "Ask for cooperation and collaboration."
- "Tell me how your suggestions will benefit the other person."

IDENTIFYING CONSEQUENCES

Before you implement assertive behaviors, it's important to identify the possible consequences of such behavior. You will need to consider the short- and long-term consequences of being assertive in situations. Decide which assertive goals seem to be worth pursuing based on the short- and long-term consequences you can identify and on an examination of your counterproductive beliefs about the situation. Go to Exercise 40 and start identifying consequences of your proposed behavior.

EXERCISE 40 Identifying Consequences

Assertiveness goal:

    Short-term consequences:

    Long-term consequences:

    Counterproductive beliefs I hold about the situation:

    Decision:

Assertiveness goal:

    Short-term consequences:

    Long-term consequences:

    Counterproductive beliefs I hold about the situation:

    Decision:

Assertiveness goal:

    Short-term consequences:

    Long-term consequences:

    Counterproductive beliefs I hold about the situation:

    Decision:

COMMUNICATING YOUR EXPECTATIONS

No one is a mind reader, but sometimes we act that way. It is not unusual to assume that other people know what you expect of them. Usually no one knows exactly what is expected of them or what to expect from others unless it is clearly stated.

If you expect others to collaborate with you, the first step toward attaining this relationship is to make a clear statement of your expectations. Some model responses for communicating expectations appear in Exercise 41.

EXERCISE 41 Being Assertive with Others

Directions: Read the situations below and see how they are handled in an assertive way. Consider modeling your responses according to the comments below or adapting the responses to your current situations.

Situation 1: Being listened to. Your colleagues or supervisor don't seem to understand or listen to you. They like you when you're positive and happy, but can't tolerate your negative feelings. You go around trying to pretend you're never angry. This time you decide to tell your colleague or supervisor what you honestly feel and that you don't expect anything but to be heard.

You: I'm upset and I want to tell you about it.
Other: Oh, gez, what now?
You: I got some bad news today and it bothered me a lot.
Other: I can tell you what I do when something like that happens to me.
You: What would be most helpful for me is if you just listen.
Other: What good is that going to do?
You: It just helps to know that you listen to and hear my feelings.
Other: Okay.
You: It would also help me a lot if you just acknowledged that you heard me say I'm angry because _____[name or relationship of other person] is hounding me again.
Other: I hear that you're angry because _____[name or relationship of other person] is hounding you again. I really know how it feels to have someone hound me.

Situation 2: Getting out of the victim or rescuer role.

Other: Why do you always _____ [complaint]."
You: I _____ [complained about action]. I do it the best way I can. If you want me to continue _____ [complained about action], please agree to let me do it the way that feels best for me.

Situation 3: Stopping sexual harassment.

Another person performs some act of sexual harassment: pinches, kisses, talks about sexual matters, etc.
You: I'd rather you didn't _____ [pinch, kiss, touch, talk about sex, etc.]. It _____ [hurts, make me feel uncomfortable].

Another use of audiotape is to record relaxing or rewarding messages. These can be saved and played back at any time you want to relax or reward yourself. A relaxation message that you can record and reuse appears in Exercise 42.

EXERCISE 42 Progressive Relaxation

Directions: Record steps 1–23 on an audiotape or ask a friend with a calm voice to do so. Either way, speak slowly, pausing for 5 seconds at each "(Pause)." If you do not have a tape recorder, find a partner to read the directions to you. Whether someone reads the material or whether you listen to a tape, be sure to find a suitable spot for relaxation, where you can be alone, where it is quiet, and where you can lie on a bed or on a soft mat on the floor. If necessary, close the door and use a Do Not Disturb sign. Remove your shoes, any binding or constricting clothing, and glasses or contact lenses. Turn off radios or television sets. Find a quiet place where the lighting is soft. If you cannot lie down, sit in a comfortable chair with your feet flat on the floor and your arms resting comfortably in your lap or by your sides.

Directions to be read into an audiotape or by your friend:

1. Close your eyes and keep them closed.
2. Pay attention to your breathing. (Pause).
3. Make sure your breathing is deep and slow and relaxed. (Pause).
4. Your breathing is smooth and effortless. (Pause).
5. When you exhale, let all the tension go out of your body. (Pause).
6. Your breathing is smooth and effortless. (Pause).
7. Now pay attention to your feet. Tighten all the muscles in your feet. Remember the sensation. Now, let your feet relax. Enjoy the sensation as your feet deeply relax. (Pause).
8. Now concentrate on your ankles and lower legs. Tighten the muscles in your ankles and lower legs. Remember the sensation. Now, let your feet relax. Enjoy the sensation as
your ankles and lower legs relax. (Pause).
9. As you exhale, let all the tension go out of your body. Tighten your knees and thighs. Remember the sensation. Now, let your knees and thighs relax. (Pause).
10. As you exhale, let all the tension go out of your body. Concentrate on breathing slowly and effortlessly. (Pause).
11. Contract the muscles of your buttocks. Remember the sensation. Now, let your buttocks relax. (Pause).
12. Now focus on your abdomen. Locate the tension in your abdomen. As you exhale, let all the tension go out of your abdomen. Your whole pelvis is relaxing. (Pause).
13. Now pay attention to your lower back. Notice where the tension is located there. As you exhale, let all the tension go out of your lower back. (Pause).
14. Your breathing is smooth and effortless. (Pause).
15. Now pay attention to your upper chest. As you exhale let all the tension go out of your chest and diaphragm. Your breathing is smooth and effortless. (Pause).

(*continued*)

EXERCISE 42 (*continued*)

16. Now pay attention to your shoulders and upper back. As you exhale, let all the tension go out of your shoulders, down your arms, and out your fingertips. (Pause).

17. When you exhale, let the tension flow out of your arms and out your fingertips. (Pause).

18. Now pay attention to your neck and throat. As you exhale, let all the tension go out of your neck and throat. Let your head bob effortlessly from side to side. Your shoulders are sinking toward your waist. Your neck is sinking toward your upper chest. (Pause).

19. As you exhale, let all the tension go out of your body. (Pause).

20. Now pay attention to your scalp. As you exhale, let all the tension go out of your scalp. Your hair is free and relaxed. Your ears are relaxed and drooping toward your shoulders. (Pause).

21. Your forehead is smooth and free from tension. Your eyelids are smooth and relaxed. As you exhale, let all the tension go out of your body. (Pause).

22. Now pay attention to your whole body. Locate any areas of tension. As you exhale, let all the tension go out of those areas. Your body is getting more and more relaxed. (Pause).

23. Note how your body feels when it is relaxed. Keep your eyes closed until you are ready to open them. When you open your eyes, you will feel relaxed and refreshed.

REFERENCES

Foster, D. G., & Marshall, M. (1994). *How can I get through to you?* New York: Hyperion.

Ramsey, G. (2002a). Law & ethics Q & A. *Nursing Spectrum Career Fitness Guide.* [On-line]. Available: www.nursingspectrum.com

Ramsey, G. (2002b). Laying down the law for nurse educators.[On-line]. Available: http://community.nursingspectrum.com/Magazine Articles/ article.cfm?AID=4889.

5

Taking and Giving Criticism

Criticism is no doubt good for the soul but we must beware that it does not upset our confidence in ourselves.

—Herbert Hoover

Taking and giving criticism assertively may not be a skill you've developed. This chapter provides information and exercises to assist you. You may not feel entirely comfortable with the idea of being critical. That may be because when you think about criticism, negative feedback is implied. You may tend to forget that criticism can be both positive ("I think you are more assertive in your tone of voice now") and negative ("Work on increasing eye contact with the other person").

If you're not used to hearing about your limitations or pointing out others' limitations or need for learning, you may feel defensive and uncomfortable with the whole evaluation process. Try to think of it as a learning process. You also have a choice. After you listen to the criticism, you can choose to implement the suggested criticism or not.

Part of your reaction to criticism probably stems from early family and school experiences. At that time, there may have been a flavor of shame or guilt whenever a parent or teacher pointed out a limitation. You also may have also felt embarrassment when a strength was discussed. Children rarely learn constructive criticism from family experiences. If you think back to your own family experiences with criticism, you will probably remember hearing a long list of shoulds and should nots. For example, "You should compliment Aunt Millie" and "You shouldn't be so messy." Some of these experiences are bound to have an impact on you if you have never had counteracting experiences that taught you how to give and take criticism comfortably.

Your educational experiences were probably not much different. If you were lucky, you may have had frequent positive evaluation conferences with an instructor who helped you identify your limitations and strengths. You may even have had an instructor who helped you learn how to decrease your limitations and enhance your strengths. Unfortunately, many evaluation conferences between teachers and students do not employ a constructive dialogue, and students frequently complain that how they are doing is a mystery to them until right before the semester ends or until they receive a grade for a course.

Even if you were fortunate enough to have received constructive feedback from instructors, you probably have not had experience in evaluating others and in providing constructive criticism for peers. You may have been taught the theory about how to provide critical evaluations, but you might not have been given practice in actually doing it. As with other skills in assertiveness, you will need to practice the components before you can expect to be expert or confident in giving and taking criticism.

A compliment is an example of positive criticism. Women seem most likely to make positive comments or evaluations. It is not uncommon for women to learn very early in their lives to use compliments to cheer someone up or to compensate for negative feelings about that person. Continuing that practice can lead to dishonesty and superficiality in social and professional relationships. Although you often may have good intentions when you compliment others, for example, merely trying to cheer them up, you run the risk of being found out. If this happens, clients or peers will not be likely to trust you. Because trust is the basis of a sound relationship, being honestly critical is very important. Women are also apt to receive "false" compliments more often because they are supposedly vain and in need of constant reassurance. Men aren't always much better in taking compliments graciously. So, whether you're male or female, taking compliments may be an area you wish to study.

Another obstacle for many men and women is the counterproductive belief that it is immodest to acknowledge a compliment and that the proper response it to protest and show embarrassment or avoid the comment. Some women and men put themselves down, often without meaning to or even being aware they are doing it.

When you are unable to acknowledge a compliment assertively, the person paying the compliment may feel uneasy for having said or done the "wrong things." If you have been in situations like this, remembered discomfort can reduce the chance that you will risk giving or taking compliments in the future.

Examine how you feel about receiving compliments or positive criticism. Some questions to ask yourself are as follows:

- Do I put myself down without meaning to?
- Can I take a compliment without denying it, giggling, or acting embarrassed?
- Can I say a simple thank-you when complimented?
- Do I feel compelled to justify or apologize for my expertise?
- Do I downplay my legitimate experience or skill?
- Do I feel obligated to return a compliment?
- Can I acknowledge a compliment?
- Do I allow myself to feel good about what I have achieved and been recognized for?

TECHNIQUES FOR TAKING AND GIVING CRITICISM

Dispel any counterproductive beliefs about giving and taking criticism. If you hold any of the following beliefs, think over how they might prevent you from being assertive and how you might go about changing your attitudes.

- If I tell others about their limitations, they will be devastated.
- I shouldn't have to tell others they are doing a good job, because they should know it.
- I don't have the right to expect others to be on time or do a competent job, especially if they have personal problems.
- I should expect more of myself than I do of others.

Acknowledging Criticism

Criticism from others can be very stressful, especially if you had parents who criticized you. Though criticism can eat at you and make you feel bad about yourself, stay hopeful. There are ways to deal effectively with criticism and come out feeling good about yourself.

Sometimes just acknowledging criticism is all that's needed. What acknowledging does is focus your energy on a positive action or clear communication. That can reduce stress and let other people know that you heard their message and are willing to discuss it. This is important because many times in a conversation the other person is unaware that critical words can affect you.

Some ways to acknowledge criticism are to say, "You're right, I did talk to the wrong person about this," or, "Yes, I didn't do the dishes." Both statements are assertive replies to criticism. Excuses and apologies aren't.

When you were little, parents and teachers might have demanded an explanation, but now you're an adult and you have the right to choose whether to give one or not. Often, it's not helpful to give an explanation because it provides more ammunition for the other person to blast you with. It also doesn't present a picture of competence and of being in charge. You may *choose* to give an explanation when someone criticizes you, but you don't have to. Remember, you are not obligated to explain yourself. It's all up to you.

Exercise 43 provides a way to prepare yourself for criticism. Please complete this exercise now.

EXERCISE 43 Identifying My Sensitivities

Directions: To prepare yourself for rejection or disapproval from others and to learn to deal with it effectively, identify your sensitivities about being rejected. Complete parts 1 and 2 below.

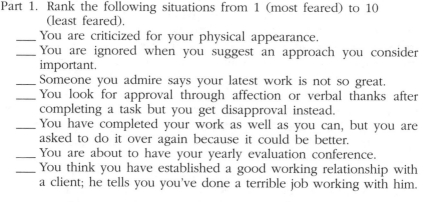

Part 1. Rank the following situations from 1 (most feared) to 10 (least feared).
____ You are criticized for your physical appearance.
____ You are ignored when you suggest an approach you consider important.
____ Someone you admire says your latest work is not so great.
____ You look for approval through affection or verbal thanks after completing a task but you get disapproval instead.
____ You have completed your work as well as you can, but you are asked to do it over again because it could be better.
____ You are about to have your yearly evaluation conference.
____ You think you have established a good working relationship with a client; he tells you you've done a terrible job working with him.

Part 2. Choose the least-feared situation and begin thinking about ways to practice overcoming your sensitivity. Some suggestions are role-playing, progressive relaxation, behavioral rehearsal. Choose one and practice overcoming your feared situation. When you feel confident dealing with that situation, move to the second least-feared situation and practice that one, then move to the next and so on.

Taking a Compliment (Positive Criticism)

Although it would seem to be a positive act to give compliments, even they can be problematic. Sometimes you may feel uncomfortable about receiving a compliment because you feel obligated to return it. There really is no reason you must give a compliment to another person just because you received one. Instead, acknowledge the compliment with a simple thank-you, and if you wish, give the other person some additional information, for example, "that's very thoughtful of you," or "I felt good when you said that."

Model Response for Taking a Compliment

Other: You really did a fine job with that report.
You: Thank you. I worked hard on it. I'm pleased you noticed my effort.

Is fear of rejection the major fear that prevents you from giving or taking criticism? If you are unsure of your identity, a minor criticism can seem devastating. As your confidence level increases through practice with the exercises in this book, you will be more able to evaluate criticism objectively. This skill can allow you to separate yourself as a person from remarks about your performance. When you cannot separate these out, you take criticism of your behavior as a frontal attack on you. Similarly, when you are nonassertive, you tend to evaluate what is said to you in terms of your own feelings of worth. When you are assertive, your self-image remains intact even when you discuss or examine your own limitations. You will learn that owning up to your strengths and limitations will earn you respect from others and yourself.

Another aspect of criticism that may be difficult for you is that it often catches you off guard. Surprises can be unsettling, but by practicing giving and taking criticism with a trusted partner, you will be more likely to apply the confidence you have developed to real-life situations.

When you are assertive, you realize that your ideas or acts may be rejected. Often, the most rejecting situations are when someone else says no to your idea, request, or action. You will probably find that the more dependent you are on others for approval, the more difficult it will be for you to hear others say no or criticize your work. You can't go through life without hearing others say no or criticizing your ideas or requests. You can make a valuable contribution even if others are critical of what you say or do. If you are assertive, you will realize that a no answer means no to a specific situation and is not a rejection of you as a person.

Sometimes other people may attempt to devalue you or convey that you are unworthy. If you are assertive, you will not accept this interpretation. At times, being assertive may mean defending yourself from attack. Just as you would not allow someone to hit you, it is important not to let others devalue you, make unfair comments about you, or put you down. Unfair criticism often relates to how the other person thinks you *should* be, and is usually unrelated to whether you accomplish your goals or not. For example, if you agree to complete a task by the end of the day and then are nagged because the task is not being completed as quickly as, or in the manner the other person wishes, you are being unfairly criticized. In this situation, the other person must either (a) verbalize the ground rules before you start, (b) recognize that you weren't given sufficient directions, admit the mistake, and give needed directions, or (c) wait until the end of the day to see if the task was completed. Complete Exercise 44 now.

EXERCISE 44 Taking Compliments

Directions: List ten of your skills that you are proud of. Find a partner and have the person compliment you on your expertise in each skill one by one. After each compliment is given, you are to say thank you, clearly, loudly, and while looking your partner in the eye. Avoid apologizing or negating your accomplishment.

Your skills:

1.

2.

3.

4.

5.

6.

7.

8.

9.

10.

Fogging

Fogging is an assertiveness technique that you can use when you receive unfair or attacking criticism. To deny the criticism would simply be responding in kind. Getting defensive or counterattacking is not useful either. The idea of fogging is to offer no resistance, yet to be persistent and independent while refusing to be manipulated. One way to do this it to agree with any truth in the other persons' statement. An example follows.

Other: You're late again. Where are you when I need you?
You: That's right. I am 5 minutes late.

Another way to use fogging is to agree with the general truth in the other person's manipulative statements:

Other: Gaining a little weight, aren't you? You know overweight is associated with heart problems and disease.
You: You're right, it is important, and when I feel the need I'll lose weight.

Fogging can help you learn to respond only to what the critic says, not to what is implied, or to what you think the criticism implies. You can use fogging in the situation in which you agreed to complete a task and then were nagged to finish.

Other: Haven't you finished yet? Sue would have finished hours ago.
You: You're right, I haven't finished yet.

Negative Assertion and Negative Inquiry

Negative assertion and *negative inquiry* are other useful techniques. Both of these approaches allow you to give an assertive, nondefensive response. You behave as if a criticism is not something to get upset about. Negative inquiry will help you to desensitize yourself to criticism so that you can listen to what you are being told, decrease others' repetitive criticism, reduce the idea that there is a strict right or wrong method of interaction, and increase the message that you can collaborate and compromise. An example of negative assertion and negative inquiry follows.

You: I've been meaning to ask you why I wasn't recommended for a promotion.
Boss: It's simple. You didn't deserve it.

You: I don't understand. What have I done that was undeserving? [negative inquiry]

Boss: You haven't been here long enough to learn the ropes.

You: Which ropes do you think I haven't learned? [negative inquiry]

Boss: You should know that you just can't speak up in a general staff meeting.

You: I guess I did make an error there. [negative assertion]

Boss: Well, as long as you know you did.

You: Anything else I can improve on?

Boss: I can't think of anything.

You: Well, I want to be recommended for the next promotion when it becomes available, so I'll learn the ropes in order to be eligible.

Assertive Probing

When criticism is used to avoid important feelings or desires, *assertive probing* can help you determine whether the criticism is constructive or manipulative. The aim of assertive probing is to clarify unclear comments.

The first step is to listen carefully to find the part of the criticism that bothers your critic. Then ask, "What is it that bothers you about that?"

Example: assertive probing

Boss: You are not doing a very good job here.

You: What is it about my work that bothers you?

Boss: You're not picking up your messages as often as you should.

You: That *is* important. I'll pick up my messages more often. Thanks for explaining the situation to me.

Broken Record

When others don't listen to your comments or accept your criticism, you can use *broken record* techniques to get their attention. You simply say it, again and again . . . and again, until you are heard. Be sure to formulate a short, specific statement that tells the other person the limits of what you'll do. Broken record resembles saying no, except the objective is different. In this case, you want the other person to accept your criticism.

Example of broken record:

You: It's important to get here on time.

Other: I would, but my car broke down.

You: Things do happen, but it's important to get here on time.
Other: I also got a terrible headache and had to stop for some aspirin.
You: Sorry to hear you had a headache, but it's important to get here on time.
Other: Okay.

Content-to-Process Shift

When the focus of the conversation drifts away from the original topic, you can use the *content-to-process shift* to help you switch from what is being discussed to what is happening between you and the other person. Some comments to use to shift from content to process include "Let's get back to what we were discussing," or "I really don't want to argue about this," or "You seem upset. What's bothering you?"

Example of content-to-process shift:

You: I wanted to talk to you about getting your work done on time.
Other: Did you know there's going to be an eclipse of the moon?
You: No, I didn't, but let's get back to what we were discussing.
Other: I really like your hair. Did you just have it cut?
You: Thanks, but we're off the point again. Let's get back to discussing your work.

Momentary Delay

You can use *momentary* delay to collect yourself and think about what you want to say next. In many situations, there is an unspoken, implied command from the other person that a statement must be answered right away. Rather than being swayed by the emotion of the moment, take a deep breath and think about your answer. There is no question that must be answered immediately unless it is a matter of life and death. Otherwise, just say, "Give me a minute to think about this." Take your time. If you can't come up with a good answer, ask for an hour, a day or even a week to come up with your answer.

Example of momentary delay:

Other: Well, what do you think about my criticism?
You: I want to answer you, but I need some time to think about it.
Other: I have to have an answer right away.
You: I realize you feel pressured to get an answer, but I want to give you the best answer I have and I need to take some time to think about it.

Time Out

When the conversation reaches an impasse, suggest a time out. This approach will only work if you set a specific time to get together to work the problem out. You might say something like "Let's sleep on this and get together tomorrow for lunch to work this out," or "I need a day to think about what you said and I suggest we get together first thing Tuesday morning to discuss it."

Deflection

This is a useful approach when you need to deflect or redirect an attack. The element of surprise, through *deflection,* can disrupt a criticism that ends in attack. Try changing the subject, by saying, for example, "Is that a new suit?" This kind of response also helps you take the criticism less seriously, thereby freeing you from stress.

Joining the Attacker

When you choose to *join the attacker,* you agree with the other person's right to experience a feeling. When you join with the attacker, you take an Aiki approach, flowing with or being the water, not the rock. A sample dialogue demonstrates the use of this technique.

Other: I'm going to have to take some action on this.
You: I don't blame you.
Other: What are you talking about, you don't blame me?
You: It's not up to me to blame anybody. I can see you're not happy, and I can't argue with that.
Other: You think you did right?
You: I guess not. You're not happy. My job is to work with you.
Other: What are you talking about?
You: Let's see if we can't work something out that we both can live with. What are some of your complaints?

Parley

This approach is most effective when you are involved in a no-win situation in which the other person is trying to make your relationship into a contest. In this case, your best response is to parley. Some comments to use are "Let's try to work out a compromise," or "Let's see if we can iron out the problem," and "If we work together, maybe we can solve both our problems."

Fighting Back

This is the best response when there is no other option, when it is a question of life or death, or the problem has a high priority. *Fighting back* means you express your anger directly and stand up to insults. Before taking any action, ask yourself the following questions:

- Does this person have nothing to lose by being aggressive? If the answer is yes, you may want to reconsider, because the other person in the interchange may not be willing to be reasonable.
- What is the minimum amount of energy I need in this situation to make my point?
- What is the best time and place for a confrontation?
- What is the best way to stop an attacker's advance?
- What is the best way to focus on the problem and not bring in personalities and generalities?
- What do I want my face and body to say and how can I be sure they say it?
- What spatial relationship to the other person is apt to end in harmony and how can I attain it?

Once you have your answers, devise your fighting-back statement. You may want to create your own comments or use on of these: "I'm angry about what you said and I'd like to talk about it," or "I feel insulted. Please don't talk to me like that. I deserve respect."

Multiple Attack

When you are attacked by several people at once, it can feel quite intimidating. If you look at the geometry of the attack, you will see that the attackers require one another to sustain the attack. Their forces create a balance when their energy is focused directly on you. Try to keep one of your attackers between you and the others, and the attack will be defused. For example, ask that person what he or she sees as the main problem and what the rest of the people there think. When family members or peers attack, it may be best to get all the attackers together. Resist becoming defensive and be sure to practice deep breathing and relaxation to keep yourself calm. Ask everyone to state their complaints clearly, and focus on your breathing while you listen.

COMMON QUESTIONS ABOUT GIVING CRITICISM

Some questions about giving criticism are asked frequently. Find the answers to some commonly asked questions below.

How do I deal with others who react defensively to my critical comments, even though my presentation is neutral or nonthreatening?

The first thing to do is to make sure your presentation of self really is neutral and nonthreatening. What may seem neutral and nonthreatening to you may not seem so to others. Record a role-play of a simple interaction that includes your critical comments. Have a neutral person listen to the tone of your voice. Or role-play a situation during which you are giving criticism and videotape it. Then do a self-critique and ask others to give you feedback on your performance.

Once you are sure you are being neutral and nonthreatening, you need to dispel some counterproductive beliefs, such as, If I am neutral and nonthreatening with criticism, others will be positive and warm. The people with whom you work probably lack skills in receiving criticism and may distort neutral messages and hear them as attacks. You will have to come to terms with this idea as well as with their right to be defensive. One way to lessen others' defensiveness is to use self-disclosure. For example, you could preface your comments with a criticism of your own performance, choosing a criticism that is accurate, so you will not be putting yourself down. A sample response might be, "I have a tough time keeping up with my report writing. That's probably why I pay attention when others don't keep up with theirs. I noticed you haven't turned in your reports for 2 weeks. I'm concerned about this and want to talk with you about it."

Another way to lessen defensiveness in others is to make your intent explicit. All communications have two levels of message: the content (this is what I'm saying), and the presentation (here is how to take what I'm saying). To make your intent explicit you might say, "I don't mean to put you down," or "I'm not saying this to make you feel uncomfortable." Sometimes such explicit statements of intent allow the other person to bear criticism in more comfort. When stating your meaning explicitly, it is crucial not to follow a statement with a put-down or attack.

Should I take different approaches in offering criticism to an authority figure, a peer, or someone over whom I have authority?

Some reality-based aspects of giving criticism to your boss is that power is involved. The degree of power varies, but it usually includes your salary and your boss's capability to deny future requests or impede your goals and power to control access to information, resources, and privileges. It may also include possession of superior knowledge. There is a tendency to grant superiors greater rights, even though their power does not invalidate your rights as a person.

There is also a tendency to relate to those both above and below us in a hierarchy as positions rather than as people. On the other hand, there may be an inclination to have too little distance from peers and to be highly competitive or fearful of criticizing them for fear of losing their support. Perhaps the most important consideration in each of these situations is not where the person is in the hierarchical structure, but whether you wish to risk the consequences of being assertive in a specific interaction with a particular person.

How do I deal with a person who has a one-track mind? No matter what approach I choose, it seems I get nowhere.

The first thing to do is to be sure you are giving "I" messages, not "you" messages, as implied by your question. Then, it is important to write specific interactions with the person, role-play them with a partner, and try to figure out where the communication went awry. After the assessment is made, an appropriate intervention or technique can be chosen.

THE PLANNED EVALUATION CONFERENCE

Whether you are evaluating another person or are being evaluated, it is helpful to think through the kinds of comments you plan to make. Constructive criticism is more apt to occur when you think through principles of effective feedback and evaluation, and practice giving and taking criticism. This will prepare you for an evaluation in assertiveness. This kind of action is called "doing your homework." If you do not do your homework and hope to deal with spontaneous situations assertively, there is less chance you will be successful. Careful planning and practice can result in feeling more confident when the actual evaluation conference occurs.

One way to do homework besides practicing through role-playing and thinking through the upcoming situation is to gather information. If you are doing an evaluation interview, have specific records that point out deficiencies or strengths and that support your point. It is useful to have written materials that you can show to, and discuss with, the other person. This creates a more objective behavior focus for discussion and decreases the chance that you or the other person will use personal attack. For example, if you wish to justify the need for more supplies, it would strengthen your case immensely if you can show a record of clients who did not receive supplies over the past month or two. Or, if you are evaluating another person who denies a deficiency, written documentation of the deficiency is more difficult for the other to deny and decreases the possibility that you will be viewed as unfair and unthinking in your criticism.

Think about ways in which you can give effective feedback. There are a number of principles of effective feedback, which are discussed as follows.

1. Feedback is effective and less threatening when you talk about behavior rather than people. For example, it is best to say, "I speak up at staff conferences," than to say, "I'm overtalkative." It is less threatening to say, "You were late five times this month," than to say, "You're a tardy person."

2. Feedback is effective when it is given in appropriate amounts, and it should be timed so the other person is ready to hear it. Giving too much information is overwhelming and will probably not be heard by the other person. Giving too little information often results in others not completely understanding where they stand. Also, feedback is effective when it focuses on a description of behavior rather than on judgments about the behavior. Try to use evaluation comments that stress performance in measurable and objective terms. Avoid using words such as *good, bad, sloppy, nosey,* and other generalizations. It is helpful to refrain from bringing up comments from past evaluation conferences. Instead, discuss specific behaviors and specific situations that are current and that can be specifically described.

3. Feedback is effective when ideas and information are shared. Encourage two-way communication and avoid giving advice. Sharing ideas and solutions encourages others to take responsibility for their actions. Telling others what to do often results in defensiveness and counterattack.

4. Feedback is effective when it deals with what is said rather than why it is said. Avoid saying, "Why didn't you?" or "Why did you?"

When you are evaluating another person or receiving an evaluation, the following actions are most apt to result in an effective evaluation and a positive change in behavior:

- The desired behaviors are clearly stated.
- The behaviors that fail to meet the level of desired behavior are stated.
- Suggestions are given for changing behavior to the desired level and are agreed on.
- There is some motivation to change behavior.
- Job descriptions are discussed until differences in interpretation are bridged.
- Each person ranks functions of the job and identifies where differences occur.
- There is agreement on when the expected behavior will be adopted.
- The other person is allowed to speak without interruption.
- Job deficiencies are discussed in detail focusing on specific behaviors.
- Facts are investigated prior to expressing an opinion.
- Responsibility is owned without blaming others.
- Before the conference is over, what has been agreed on is summarized.

Some common errors in evaluation interviews that you need to watch for are attacking others' attitude, trying to convince others to change their attitude, allowing the evaluation to be a social visit, getting into a charge-excuse cycle, and going over points that have already been made repeatedly.

Two model responses for evaluation conferences follow.

Model Response

You: I want to talk with you about your work. [purpose is stated] Let's look at the job description and identify where we agree and disagree about your performance. [suggests collaboration and two-way communication]

Other: [Pointing to job description] I think I write good reports, but I need to work on talking to clients. [states a specific strength and a limitation]

You: I agree with you about needing to learn better communication skills, but I disagree about your reports. [disagrees without attacking] Did you bring two samples of your reports with you? [has done homework and planned for the evaluation]

Other: Yes, here they are. I think they cover everything. [gives "I" messages and evaluates behavior]

You: Let's look at this one. Although the report is neat and clearly written, it's missing an introduction and summary. There are no comments about what information you gave the client. I think these are important components of reports. [points to specific deficiencies]

Other: You're right. I overlooked that. I will try to remember to include those components in my next reports. [owns up to error and maintains two-way communication]

You: How can we plan so that those important aspects appear in your next report?

Other: I can ask Trudy to look over my reports before I hand them in. [suggestions for changing behavior are stated]

You: That sounds like a plan. Let's agree on a date for reevaluation of this aspect.

Other: How about 2 weeks?

You: Fine.

Model Response

You: I want to talk with you about your work. It is important that clients be seen when they get to the office. I have a copy of your job description. Let's look at it together. [points out deficiency and suggests collaboration and two-way evaluation]

Other: My union says I don't have to do that! [Uses a subtle threat: I will call the union in]

You: This is a copy of the latest job description agreed on between the union and management. [has done homework and obtained job description]

Other: That's not my job. [denies responsibility]

You: This is a copy of your job description. I expect you to follow it. [broken-record technique; states desired behavior]

Other: No one else does. [avoids taking responsibility for own action]

You: We're talking about you now. [sticks to issue]

Other: What do you want from me?

You: I want you to be available when your client arrives. [states desired behavior]

Other: I don't know why you pick on me. [guilt induction]

You: This is your evaluation. It's my job to work with you to be sure you complete your work. What happens that you aren't available when your client arrives? [obtains information before suggestion a solution]

Other: Sometimes your assistant asks me to do things around the office.

You: I will talk to my assistant about that and work it out with him so he doesn't ask you to do work for him when you already have an assignment.

Other: I only do what he tells me to do.
You: I want you to be able to complete your assignment. I'd like to talk with you in 2 weeks to see how you are doing with this part of your assignment.
Other: Okay.
You: Good, then we're agreed to meet again in 2 weeks for a reevaluation of your work. [summarizes]

Go now to Exercise 45 for ways to practice taking and giving criticism.

EXERCISE 45 Practice for Giving and Taking Criticism

Directions: Each situation that follows is labeled with the type of behavior required. Not all comments by other people in the situations are assertive. It is your task to use assertive comments. Practice writing and saying a response to each situation until you feel comfortable with it. Then move on to the next one. When you have mastered all practice situations, design your own situations for practice. Be sure to identify real-life situations to use as homework assignments.

Situation 1: Taking Compliments

You shared your opinion in a work conference. You feel good about your accomplishment. You know that your supervisor sometimes gives left-handed compliments. You want to take the compliment without responding to supervisor's fear.

Supervisor: You really spoke up in there. Do you think they'll be mad?
You: _____

_____

Supervisor: A couple of them looked pretty upset.
You: _____

_____

Situation 2. Praising Others

You want to let a colleague know that you think she or he is doing a fine job.
You: _____

Coworker: Oh, it was nothing.
You: _____

_____

Situation 3: Owning up to Mistakes

You know you forgot to complete a work task. When you finally get to talk to your client, he's quite angry.

(continued)

Client: Where have you been? I needed your help.
You: _____

             _____

Client: Don't give me excuses. I'm a client here and I expect to be
             treated right.
You: _____

             _____

Situation 4: Pointing Out Others' Limitations

You have planned a conference to discuss the performance of one of
       your supervisees. This employee has difficulty setting pri-
       orities and never completes work on time.
You: _____

Supervisee: I always get my work done, don't I?
You: _____

             _____

Supervisee: The trouble is I have more difficult clients than anyone
             else has.
You: _____

             _____

6
Time Management Skills

Lost time is never found again.

—Benjamin Franklin

Managing time effectively can be an important stress reducer. This chapter provides steps to follow to enhance your time management skills.

Are you having difficulty completing tasks? Do you feel overwhelmed by demands and details? Do you chronically miss deadlines? Do you rush around fatigued, or have hours of nonproductive activity? Do you have insufficient time for rest or personal relationships? If you answered yes to one or more of these questions, you could benefit from time management procedures.

The first step in effective time management is exploring how time is currently being spent. An easy way to do this is to divide the day into three segments: waking through lunch, end of lunch through dinner, and end of dinner until bedtime. Carry a small notebook and write down the number of minutes you spend for each activity in each time segment. Keep the inventory for 3 days. At the end of the time, examine the total amount of time you spend in various activities.

Table 6.1 provides a time management assessment for one person. Take a look at Table 6.1 now and see how to set up your time management inventory. Based on a review of the inventory, the following decisions were made:

1. Put out clothes for the next day prior to going to bed.
2. Get up at the alarm and limit shower to 5 minutes.
3. Make breakfasts that don't require cooking, cut dinner preparation to 30 minutes, and enlist family to do food preparation 3 days a week.
4. Ask for a late lunch to take advantage of most productive work hours (11 A.M. to 2 P.M.).

TABLE 6.1 Time Management Assessment

Activity	Time in mins	Activity	Time in mins
Waking through lunch		*After lunch through dinner*	
Lying in bed and thinking	20	Working with clients	90
Showering	20	Daydreaming	20
Deciding what to wear	25	Working on report	20
Cooking breakfast	15	Talking and socializing	30
Reading paper and eating	30	Commuting	30
Commuting to work	30	Shopping	45
Routine paperwork	30	Phone calls	30
Daydreaming	10	Cooking	90
Nonmandatory meeting	60	Eating	30
Working with clients	120	*After dinner until retiring*	
Lunch	45	Phone calls	60
		TV	90
		Studying	90
		Preparing for bed/reading	30

5. Use thought-stopping to limit daydreaming.
6. Stop attending nonmandatory, nonproductive meetings.

The next step is to set priorities. Begin by making a list of things you most want to accomplish in the near future and compare it to how you now spend your time. Visualize yourself being told you have 6 months to live and imagine how you will best spend the time. Make the list without stopping to evaluate or judge what you write.

Next, make a list of l-month and l-year goals you believe you can reasonably accomplish in terms of work, improvement, and recreation. Then sit back and reflect on long-, medium- and short-term goals. Next, prioritize each list by deciding which are top-drawer items (most essential or desired), middle-drawer items (can be put off for a while, but still important), and bottom drawer (can easily be put off indefinitely with no harm done).

Here are some examples of time management goals:

1. Buy a new car (l-year goal).
2. Write an article for a journal (lifetime goal: to contribute to the profession.)
3. Have dinner out with husband once a week (l-month goal).

4. Investigate ways of becoming a consultant (lifetime goal: to communicate my knowledge).
5. Take dance lessons with my husband (1-year goal).
6. Complete old records file at work (1–month goal).

If you feel overwhelmed by any of the goals, you can break them down into manageable steps. For example, the goal of investigating ways of becoming a consultant could be divided into the following steps:

1. Borrow a friend's book on consultation and read a chapter a week.
2. Talk with other people who are consultants and ask one or more to be my mentor.
3. Make a list of my knowledge and my marketable consulting skills.
4. Purchase stationery and business cards and develop a brochure detailing my consulting skills.
5. Send out a query letter to potential clients, using my stationery, business cards, and brochures.

If you find it difficult to get started even after breaking down your priorities into manageable steps that you can develop a daily To Do list including everything you want to accomplish that day. Rate each item top, middle, or bottom priority and work only on the top priority items for the day.

Here are some other tips for making more time.

- Learn to say no. Remind yourself, This is my life and my time to spend doing what best suits me. Only when your boss asks should you spend time on low-priority items. Be prepared to say "I don't have the time." If necessary, take an assertiveness training course.
- Build time into your schedule for unscheduled events, interruptions, and unforeseen occurrences.
- Keep a list of short, 5–minute tasks that can be done any time you are waiting or are between other tasks.
- Learn to do two tasks at once: plan dinner while driving home or organize an important letter or list while waiting in line at the grocery store.
- Delegate bottom-drawer tasks to sons, daughters, spouses, secretaries, or in-laws.

- Get up 15 to 30 minutes earlier every day.
- Allow no more than 1 hour of TV watching per day. Use TV as a reward for working on your top-drawer items.

Part of time management is the ability to make decisions. Procrastination is a great time robber. Here are some tips for overcoming procrastination:

1. Analyze the costs and risks of delay.
2. Examine the payoffs you receive from procrastinating (avoiding facing failure, others take care of you, you get attention if you're chronically unhappy).
3. Exaggerate and intensify whatever you are doing to put off the decision. When you are thoroughly bored, the decision may seem more attractive than whatever you're doing to procrastinate.
4. Write down how long each delay takes.
5. To make unimportant decisions, flip a coin, choose south or east over north or west; pick left over right, smooth over rough, shortest over longest, closest over farthest away, or the one that comes first alphabetically.
6. Take baby steps toward the decision, for example, if you want to decide to repair a dress, take out the thread and needle and place them by you as a lead-in to the decision to begin.
7. Avoid beginning a new task until you have completed a predetermined segment of the current one. Allow yourself to experience fully the reward of finishing something, a payoff of decision making.

Here are some quick tips for reducing stress:

- Get up half an hour earlier in the morning for a hassle-free start to your day.
- Break down tasks into steps; you'll feel less pressured to get things done when you focus on one small step at a time.
- Exercise everyday to prevent stress build-up. Take an exercise break instead of a coffee break if your work is stressing you.
- Set realistic daily goals and remind yourself that you'll probably never achieve them all and that's okay.
- Identify one thing you like to do and make sure you do it regularly.
- Shorten waiting times by bringing along something you enjoy: needlepoint, knitting, a good book, or some other activity that makes you feel good about yourself.

- When an accident or mishap occurs, take a time out and tell yourself that mistakes happen and you're not perfect and you can't control everything so you might as well accept it. You might even try to laugh at your shortcomings. It will put the event in perspective.

7

Managing Anger

Every stroke our lung strikes is sure to hit ourselves at last.
—William Penn

Everyone experiences anger. Assertive skills can help you handle anger and teach others to handle theirs. For many people the most anxiety-provoking situation they face is dealing with anger—whether their own or someone else's. It is easy to recognize assertive anger because it is direct and openly stated. It is not physically or verbally abusive and respects the other person's rights.

Societal prohibitions exist about releasing anger in a direct way. Many professionals are taught never to get angry with their clients or supervisors—or at least not to show it. This practice leads to high anxiety and fear about dealing with anger.

You probably operate in a work or family system that perpetuates myths about what can and cannot be achieved. When you buy into these myths, you may experience anger because of unrealistic expectations that have been set. If you deny yourself or allow others to trample on your rights, it can lead to feeling ill, being overly critical of others, making more mistakes than usual, or crying or taking your frustrations out on others.

Acknowledge that you are a human being who has all the same emotions and experiences as other people, including anger. You have the right to feel your own unique and special qualities, to express both joy and anger, to be accepted as a person of worth and dignity, to have access to help and support, to make choices and decisions, and to have a degree of privacy.

To deal with anger effectively, it is important to identify and dispel any counterproductive beliefs you have about expressing or dealing with anger such as:

- I shouldn't get angry with a client or family member.
- I might explode or harm someone if I express my anger.

- I don't want to antagonize coworkers or clients, because I can't handle their anger.
- If others see me angry, they'll think I'm irrational or ill-tempered.
- If I express my anger, the other person will fall apart.

Dealing with other people's anger may be easier for you than dealing with your own. When a client, coworker or family member yells or shouts at you, the important thing to remember is to wait until that person calms down. There is no way to reason with someone who is out of control. Besides, you might lose your temper as well. Some comments to use are "I hear your anger," "Loud voices won't solve this, please lower your voice," and "I'd like to work this out, but I can't when I'm shouted at."

These comments are especially effective when spoken in a soft voice. It is difficult for others to maintain their anger indefinitely without fuel from you. Reflect back what the other person is saying, which often calms things down. Or if you find the anger is increasing your anxiety, you can leave the angry person and say, "I can't talk now, but I want to settle this later." This approach will leave the channels of communication open and will allow you to resume the discussion later on. Also, if no one is listening to the other, you might as well break off the discussion and resume it later.

Although it may be difficult for you to be comfortable about expressing your anger, it is important for a number of reasons. First, if you don't express anger, you will convert it into depression, headache, or problems with other body systems, or you will add it to other angers until it builds up and you explode in rage. Neither result is healthy for you. Second, you have the right to express yourself, including your anger. Third, clients and coworkers and family members can learn to deal with anger appropriately by watching you deal with yours. Acting as if others cannot learn to deal with their own and others' anger is overprotective and denies their right to learn to deal with feelings effectively. By serving as a role model for others, you can be a health-enhancing person.

The first step in dealing with your anger is to recognize and experience it. Once you realize your anger is manageable, it will be easier for you to experience it without fear. Complete Exercise 46 now.

EXERCISE 46 Structured Release of Anger

Directions: Find a partner. Switch roles after you have completed the steps and help your partner practice. Both of you should read the directions for partner before attempting the exercise. Before practicing, get a hand mirror that is large enough for you to see your face and expressions easily.

1.   Directions for partner: Your task is to help your partner learn how to convey some aspects of verbal and nonverbal anger in an authentic and comfortable way. To complete this task, it is important that you direct your partner to do each task until both of you are satisfied with the outcome. Be sure to give feedback, such as "Say that again only this time sound angry."

2.   Now complete the following steps until you both agree you are satisfied with the outcome. Don't rush. This exercise takes time to produce results. Read steps a, b, and c out loud to your partner. Be sure to use a mirror when it's called for.

Step a.   "Close your eyes and picture a situation in which you felt angry. Remember who was there, what was said, and how you felt. Actually picture yourself in that situation. Make a mental picture of yourself in your anger. Do you have that picture?" (If not, coach your partner until that picture is clear, for example, "take your time and enlarge that situation in your mind.")

Step b.   "Open your eyes and look at your face in the mirror. Does it look different? Are you showing the anger on your face that you felt during the situation?" (Give feedback about whether your partner looks angry. Show anger on your face by wrinkling your forehead and glaring with your eyes. Ask your partner to imitate you. Experiment with how your face and your partner's face can show anger.)

Step c.   Ask your partner to say, "I'm really angry [mad, pissed off, etc.] in an angry tone of voice while looking in the mirror. Choose the words you use when angry and say them into the mirror using an appropriate tone of voice and facial expression." (Make helpful comments to your partner, e.g., "Sound more angry," "Say it as if you mean it."

TRANSFORMING ANGER INTO PROBLEM-SOLVING

Although it is assertive to express anger directly, it is also useful to transform anger into problem-solving action. Most of us have been taught by our parents to comply. If we hadn't, families would be in chaos with all family members going their own way. It's simply just more efficient for a family to be run like a totalitarian regime, at least when we're babies. Parents probably get into a pattern and forget that as their children get older, they are perfectly capable of, and even need practice in, learning to make good decisions. But teaching and learning decision-making takes time, commitment, and effort. In the short run, it may seem better for parents to just make the decisions. In the long run this leads to a society of people who have never learned how to make constructive decisions and have no idea how to teach others to make them.

In school, compliance is also rewarded. Again, the chaos factor is involved. All children in a given school cannot all be making independent decisions about everything or daily activities would never get done. (Although it has never been researched, it might be a good experiment to see if students who are provided with problem-solving skills and then are allowed to make their own decisions don't mature more quickly and turn into better citizens.)

At work, compliance is also rewarded. Bosses and leaders want their egos massaged and want things done efficiently. Often, they don't stop to think that their employees would do more work and be a lot more satisfied if they were involved in decision-making.

Problem-solving requires a take-charge attitude. The following are specific steps that must be taken to problem-solve:

1. Define the problem. Make sure you do this in very precise terms. Problems can seem overwhelming when they're vague. For example, saying "I hate my job" is general. So is "My boss expects too much and that stresses me." You have to define what you hate about your job or what your boss expects more specifically if you want to come up with a solution. Ask yourself, What exactly do I hate about my job? Specific problem statements include "I hate that I have to do everyone else's work and when I get behind my skin breaks out," or "I hate that when I have to write a report I feel stressed and I take tranquilizers." The difference between a specific statement and a vague one is that when the problem is stated specifically, it leads you to what you have to do to find a solution. (In the first example above, you have to change the environment so that you're not doing everyone else's work or you have to reduce your stress so that your skin won't break out.)

2. Brainstorm a solution. The next step in problem solving is finding a solution. Ask yourself, What has to happen so that this problem is no longer a problem? Begin to think about possible solutions. Rule out none of them yet. That's what brainstorming is all about—just letting the ideas flow. Don't worry about whether they make sense; just write them down as they come to mind, even if some of them sound silly or fantastic. Once you have them all written down, it is time to decide which ones will work. Rate them from 1 (could work) to 4 (no way). Once you've rated them, focus on those you've numbered with a 1. Decide which one has the very best chance of being successful. Remember, no solution is 100% surefire. Choose the one that has the best chance of solving the problem.

3. Take action. If your action involves speaking to someone, practice what you're going to say before speaking. You can record it and then rate yourself on how convincing you sound or look. Keep in mind that if the problem has a long history, it may not be solved in one short discussion. Think about laying the groundwork with the initial discussion.

TRANSFORMING YOUR ANGER INTO OTHER POSITIVE ACTIONS

Anger is a normal feeling. Don't avoid it, just learn to transform it into positive action. Here are some ideas for doing just that.

Use An Anger Journal

One of the best methods for directing anger in or out is the Anger Journal (McKay, Rogers, & McKay, 1995). You can begin to change your anger, but first you have to identify what proceeds it.

Purchase a journal that suits you, one you feel good about writing in. For the next week, write in your Anger Journal each time you feel angry. You may be too upset to write right away, but go back and reconstruct what led up to your anger. While you're writing in your journal, focus on four questions:

1. What stresses came before my anger? Think about what you were feeling or experiencing prior to anger. Did you feel anxious, hurt, sad, or guilty? Did you experience frustration, threat or any uncomfortable sensations? Write down anything you can remember.

2. What thoughts triggered your anger? Think back to exactly what you were thinking at the moment you became aware of your anger. A common trigger is a sentence with the word "should" in it, which carries the implication that you or others must admit wrongdoing. Triggers also carry harmful intent as if whoever did this did it to you and did it with intent to harm. As you begin to separate out these "shoulds" and "shouldn'ts" you can begin to understand what triggers your anger and identify the point at which these thoughts turn from stress into anger.

3. What were my feelings right before the trigger statements took over? It's not easy to separate your anger from your trigger statements, but it will be very helpful if you can. It will help you move out of the victim role and into empowerment.

4. Did my anger block stress or discharge anger? Did you feel better, if only for a few moments after you got angry? Even though the relief is short-lived, it reinforces the idea in your mind that venting your anger is useful.

Use Imagery to Transform Anger

If anger gets in your way, use one of the methods below to feel better and get your focus back.

Method 1:

1. Close your eyes and identify where in your body the anger resides. Is there anger in your heart? your stomach? your neck? your back? someplace else?
2. Collect all the anger from where it is.
3. Using your imagination, put the anger in an some kind of container; whatever type you visualize is fine.
4. Close the lid of the container.
5. Lock the container and throw away the key.
6. Send it somewhere far, far away where it can no longer influence you.

Method 2:

1. Close your eyes.
2. Turn your anger into a color.
3. Turn the color into a liquid.
4. Let all the anger drain out of your fingers and toes.
5. Let the anger drain onto the floor, out the door, and far, far away.

Use Written Methods to Transform Anger

There are several ways you can use written methods to reduce anger. One method is to write a letter that explains the hurts that cause the anger. The letter need not be sent, in fact, it may be better if it is not. The purpose of the letter is to help you identify and verbalize your anger and its source. Next, you can write a letter of forgiveness, forgiving the other person for their part in your anger. Finally, if you feel you express anger in poorly controlled ways, write a letter to yourself. The purpose of this letter is to forgive yourself for expressing anger or losing control.

Use Drawing to Transform Anger

Collect some colored pens or crayons and some drawing paper. Sit down in a quiet spot and draw the following situations:

- You discharging all your anger
- You looking healthy and calm
- Draw yourself in your perfect job

Transform Angry Self-Talk

We talk to ourselves in our head. A lot of what is said up there is angry, self- or other-deprecating, and generally nonconstructive. Some of this discussion is just a replaying of old tapes we learned in our families. Maybe Dad put down Mom or Sis put down Brother or vice versa. After you hear anything long enough, it becomes ingrained, especially if you're young, without power and impressionable. Although you may not think so, this angry self-talk influences you and your behavior. You may even hear yourself saying something your mother, father, or some other family member said to you.

Your job, if you want to rid yourself of angry self-talk, is to begin to identify it. Listen to what you're saying to yourself. When you hear an angry comment that is critical of yourself or others, stop it in the middle and say to yourself, "Cancel that thought." You might also consider replacing negative and angry self-talk with positive and uplifting self-talk. Some examples appear below:

Angry self-talk	Positive self-talk
That was a stupid thing to do.	I'm allowed to make mistakes.
That man just cut me off. How dare he?	I'll drive defensively and make sure I'm safe.

I'll never amount to anything. They're just idiots and incompetents.	I'm already a caring human being. Everybody functions at the highest level possible; I'll send them some positive energy to help them function at a higher level.

LEARNING FORGIVENESS

It's hard to imagine going through life without being treated unfairly. Is forgiveness an issue for you? Are you looking for a way to dissolve those sad or mad feelings toward somebody who hurt you?

What Forgiveness Is

Forgiveness means deciding not to punish the accused, to take action on that decision, and then to fully experience the emotional relief that brings. Forgiveness means you have at least three choices: reconciliation; easing your conscience and letting go of any guilt about not forgiving; freedom from anger and resentment.

Benefits of Forgiveness

What are the benefits of forgiving someone else? For one thing, it will be good for your health. An angry heart can't be a healthy one. You don't want this hurt to eat away at you. It can harm your immune system and make your friends and family keep out of your way.

If you forgive, you'll have warmer relationships with other people and yourself (building your self-esteem). You will experience a calm in this otherwise violent world. You will no longer be under the power of the one who wronged you because you won't be angry or obsessing about whether to forgive that person or not. You'll be released from the destructiveness that vengeance perpetuates. The offender will also experience relief. There will be an increase in the flow of love—something there can't be too much of in this troubled world—and maybe even love for the one who wronged you (Affinito, 1999).

Look at it this way: You have the most to gain from being the forgiver. It is almost a selfish act.

Beginning Steps Toward Forgiveness

What do you do to gain self-control so you can forgive?

1. Get in touch with your own sense of morality and standards for human contact. What do you expect of others and of yourself?
2. Identify any failure on your part to live up to your own standards.
3. Either lower your standards to come into line with your behavior or make your thoughts more positive and your behavior more forgiving.
4. Set a goal of recovering from any hurt you feel due to the other person's offense.
5. Get a grip on the concept of justice and your part in bringing it about.
6. Take a problem-solving approach, coaching yourself to believe that you can figure out how to forgive, make the necessary changes, take the necessary steps and end up feeling good about yourself and others.

Identify Obstacles to Forgiveness

Certain feelings can interfere with your attempts to forgive. The most prominent ones are shame, blame, and guilt.

Shame

Healthy shame, also called humility, brings you in touch with your own imperfections. It can help you avoid the pitfall of seeing everything in terms of black and white, good and bad. It can help you decide which hurts can be fixed and which can't be. When you're humble, you realize that it's only human to make mistakes and you won't get caught in the trap of always trying to be right. Complete Exercise 47 now.

EXERCISE 47 Healthy Shame

Directions: Check off the items below if you believe they are true.

___ I realize I make mistakes, too.
___ I am willing to face my failures openly and honestly.
___ I can accept that I can never know exactly why another person did anything.
___ I can let go of good or bad comparisons between me and other people.
___ I have faith in my own moral standards.
___ I accept that no solution is ever perfect or final.
___ I know that along with my failings, I have positive traits that make me a complete person.
___ I admit that I don't always live up to my own standards, but I try to.
___ I focus on me, not on the wrongdoing of the other person, when trying to fix a relationship.
___ I realize that the journey toward self-knowledge is ongoing.
___ I accept that no one is always right.
___ I give myself permission to be flexible and consider situational morality.
___ I can say "I'm ashamed" and still feel good about myself.

The more items you checked, the more reason you have to believe you have healthy shame. Congratulations! It will serve you well.

You need healthy shame to work toward forgiveness. Without it, you cannot bring morality and past knowledge into play in your decision making. Once you gain some emotional distance from the wrong, you can use healthy shame to allow yourself to identify when you were not always morally correct.

Toxic shame feels awful and leads you to irrational interpretation and maybe even depression because it is often expressed as worthlessness, inferiority, and the need to hide your true self. Many small (and sometimes large) situations contribute to toxic shame. It all starts in childhood when we, not our deeds, are criticized. It's then we start to believe that we are bad people. Everybody has some toxic shame. To forgive, you need to identify and accept your toxic shame and not let it cloud your decision making (Bradshaw, 1988).

Our culture contributes to toxic shame. If you buy into the success ethic, your toxic shame will increase. This ethic says you will succeed against tremendous odds, if only you try. Because only a few do succeed in this way, it paves the way for the rest of us to feel inadequate and thereby shamed.

Our culture also holds to the individual ethic, that you must stand out and be different. It also holds the opposite ethic that it's important to be sociable and well-liked and not stand out too much.

Our culture also encourages us to be independent and self-sufficient. If you follow this injunction, you can wind up feeling awfully alone and isolated. People need people in order to be healthy.

If you hold any of these ethics, you may suffer terrible toxic shame. This is in addition to any physical, emotional, or sexual abuse you may have suffered or witnessed and any humiliation you endured as a method of discipline. If this is the case with you, start to get clear on just whose behavior was truly shameful: it wasn't yours.

Sometimes toxic shame is so painful you don't even allow yourself to know about it. Still, there are some clues that you may be suffering from toxic shame. Go to Exercise 48 now and examine your sources of toxic shame.

EXERCISE 48 Toxic Shame

Directions: Check off the items you agree with.

___ I'm afraid to reveal myself to anyone for fear they won't like what they find out.

___ I believe only I am lacking in self-control and self-knowledge.

___ I am more concerned with what other people think than in trusting my own sense of who I am and what I want.

___ I believe I have to be right 100% of the time or I'm totally wrong.

___ I feel too emotionally involved in revenge or other negative feelings to focus my energy on a problem-solving approach to my difficulties.

___ I believe I am basically flawed and my positive traits can never make up for that fact, and I live in dread that someone will find out.

___ I'm afraid to try problem-solving for fear that my solution won't be perfect so that by a process of elimination, it will be worthless.

___ I see myself and everyone else as either totally right or totally wrong.

___ I hold on to a sense of morality someone else taught me without examining whether it's right for me.

___ I cannot admit it when I'm ashamed because it would be too painful.

Count up the items you checked. The more checks, the more toxic shame you hold and the more it can hold you back from forgiving others and yourself.

Blame

A good way to avoid shame is to blame someone else. Although this can reduce your shame, it also makes it difficult for you to reduce it. Blaming someone else is almost second nature when you've been hurt. On the other hand, you might be one of the people who is reluctant to blame others no matter what. This can also lead to a less than helpful solution. In this case, by not holding the other person responsible for his or her part in the problem, your healing can be blocked.

Guilt

Guilt is appropriate when you've violated moral standards. Lack of guilt can reflect a lack of conscience and allow you to do things that might harm other people. Inappropriate guilt can get in the way of forgiveness because you may blame yourself for invalid reasons. Examine your guilt to see if it's appropriate, looking for possible causes for your self-punishing behavior. If you find yourself feeling guilty but don't know why, you may have tapped into some toxic shame.

Grief

Grief is probably part of what you're experiencing. If you've been offended, you've lost something and grief is natural reaction to it. You will need to grieve for what was lost in order to move on and forgive.

First, you will need to separate out your anger, your shame, and your guilt. Only then can you grieve unencumbered.

Journal writing is a good tool for this purpose. Purchase a journal that pleases you and begin to write in it. Write at least a page, giving specific examples whenever you can, on your own evaluation and understanding of the following:

1. Your healthy shame versus your toxic shame
2. Your appropriate blame versus your inappropriate blame
3. Your appropriate guilt versus your inappropriate guilt
4. Your grief that is distinguished and clear versus grief that is confused and bundled with other feelings.

Use the following affirmations to help you develop a forgiving attitude; say each one 20 times a day and write them on 3 x 5 cards and put them in prominent spots where you will read them often:

- I can understand and get past the hurt I feel.
- I can use the energy from my anger and resentment to help me find creative ways to express my forgiveness.
- I can reestablish a relationship that's right for me with people who have offended me.
- When bad things happen to me I can keep calm and stay strong.
- I can take responsibility for what I say and do, and feel good about it.
- I can be around people who have offended me and stay calm and peaceful.
- I can talk about past hurts with people who have hurt me and remain calm and clear.
- I appreciate myself and my life.
- My conscience is clear and I am living my values.

Catastrophizing Thoughts

Catastrophizing thoughts can make things seem worse than they are. Some examples of catastrophizing thoughts are *This is the worst thing that's ever happened to me; I can't stand the way I've been treated; This is terrible; This is awful.*

Once you start having catastrophizing thoughts, it is difficult to be forgiving. To get yourself back to a calmer focus, tell yourself *This is frustrating, but it's not the end of the world; Getting all upset isn't going to help; There's no guarantee that I'll get what I want, but that's no reason not to stay calm.*

Demanding/Coercing Thoughts

Demanding/coercing thoughts tend to turn your wants into demands. It is the tendency to think that things *should, ought, need to be, have to, must be* certain ways. When you demand that people react in a certain way, anger, not forgiveness can result. Examples of demanding/coercing thoughts are *She shouldn't have hurt my feelings; This isn't fair.*

Helpful thoughts can counter demanding/coercing thoughts. Some examples are *I can't always expect people to act the way I want them to; Things don't always have to be done my way; I'm going to handle this by focusing on it as a problem to be solved.*

Overgeneralized Thoughts

When you overgeneralize, you go way beyond the facts to make things seem much bigger than they really are. By blowing the situation out of proportion, you only make yourself more angry, not more forgiving. Examples of overgeneralized thoughts are *I'll never trust anyone again; I'm never going to get over this.*

When you find yourself using overgeneralized thinking, use self-thoughts that reduce overgeneralization. *In the greater scheme of things, this is not that important; This is a negative happening, but I can handle it; There is no need to get all upset about this.*

Categorical Thinking

When you label situations in extreme, deprecating terms, you're using categorical thinking. Examples of categorical thinking are *What a jerk! He's worthless; She's no good.* These kind of thoughts just crank up your anger and make forgiveness impossible.

Some thoughts to counter categorical thinking with are *Cancel that; she's just somebody I disagree with. This is bad, but it can be fixed.*

One-track Thinking

When you think things can only go one way and you personalize the reasons rather than identifying multiple reasons for why things happened, you're using one-track thinking. If you use this type of thinking, your anger will rise. Here are some one-track thoughts: *She wouldn't have done that if she was my friend; He's doing this just to get to me.*

Sometimes you could be right, but it only leads to more frustration and anger, so it probably isn't worth it to pursue this line of thinking. Instead, use helpful self-thoughts to reduce one-track thinking: *I'm not going to jump to conclusions. I'll check out the facts first; I may not have all the facts, but I'm going to get them; Getting so angry will not help me figure out what went wrong.*

REFERENCES

Bradshaw, J. (1988). *Healing the shame that binds you.* Deerfield Beach, FL: Health Communications.

McKay, M., Rogers, P. D, & McKay, J. (1995). *When anger hurts. Quieting the storm within.* Oakland, CA: New Harbinger.

8
Accepting Your Power to Heal and Be Healed

You must be the change you wish to see happen in the world.
—Mahatma Ghandi

Accepting your power to heal and be healed includes discrete behaviors. You must first accept that you deserve to be healed. Once you've accomplished that, you can move on to using stress management to heal, to expressing your anger directly, to transforming your anger to problem-solving, to seeking forgiveness, and to what leaders can do to heal and be healed.

YOU DESERVE TO BE HEALED

You may not believe it yet, but you deserve to be healed. Once you've reached acceptance, you can begin to use stress management to heal, to use problem-solving instead of anger, to transform your anger, to learn forgiveness, and—if you're a leader—take action to help heal your employees (see Table 8.1).

USING STRESS MANAGEMENT TO HEAL

No matter how many techniques or procedures you learn for being assertive, you will not use them often if you feel highly anxious or fearful. At times you may choose to avoid making assertive statements rather than experience the discomfort of anxiety that follows. Also, if you are highly anxious, you will usually communicate this to others, and your verbally assertive message may be missed because your listeners are paying more attention to your discomfort.

TABLE 8.1 You Deserve to Be Healed

Directions: Read the following treatment aloud at least once a day. If you wish, record it on an audiotape and play it when you get up and when you go to bed each day.

I deserve to be healed. Not just part of me, but all of me. I now move past negative feelings, thoughts, and relationships. I release and let go of the limitations of my family, friends, colleagues, and work settings. I love them all, and I go beyond them. I am not negative or limiting beliefs. I am not bound by any fears or prejudices. I no longer identify with limitation in any shape or form.

No matter what happens around me, in my mind I am totally free. I now move into a new consciousness, a place where I am willing to see myself and others differently. I am willing to create a new reality, new thoughts about myself and others, a new life. My new thinking becomes my experience.

I now know and affirm that I am one with the power of the Universe. As a result, I now prosper in many ways. The totality of all possibilities lies before me. I deserve to be healthy, wealthy and safe. I deserve a long history of joy and happiness. I accept the freedom to be.

The Universe is willing to manifest my new beliefs, which will affect many others. I accept this abundance with joy, pleasure, and gratitude. I realize now that I am deserving of all good. I accept all positives that now will come to me and agree to share them with everyone around me.

Anxiety often has a contagious aspect. If you are anxious, others may often sense this on some level of awareness and will become more tense themselves. If you are relaxed, there is a greater likelihood that those around you will be relaxed and that you will be more open and able to listen to them. Being relaxed decreases the sense of threat in a situation, which allows you to discuss issues that would lead to avoidance or aggression if the atmosphere were more tense. For these reasons, it is wise to learn and systematically practice techniques to decrease your anxiety and fear.

You can use thought stoppage, systematic desensitization, affirmations, guided imagery, and self-coaching to heal yourself. Two other approaches—dealing with anger and handling backlash—will assist in the healing process. If time constraints are increasing your anxiety and stress, try time management procedures.

Thought Stoppage

Thought stoppage is a behavioral procedure that requires effort and systematic practice. Use this procedure when you have self-defeating thoughts that prohibit you from acting assertively. Some self-defeating thoughts are "I can't do this," "I can't stand this, If I'm assertive, it won't work, I'm not any good," "I' can't complete my work on time," "I'm stupid."

Exercise 49 can give you practice with thought stoppage. The procedure can teach you to put an end to self-defeating thoughts by saying "Stop!" whenever a self-defeating thought comes to mind and then following that act with a period of conscious relaxation. The procedure requires that you use this method each time you have a self-defeating thought, or the method will not work. At first, there may be an increase in self-defeating thoughts because you are focusing on them. This is normal. As you continue to use the procedure, you will gain control over those thoughts. Meanwhile, the frequency of self-defeating thoughts will drop off. Even after you master this procedure, self-defeating thoughts may emerge during times of stress. Continue to use the "Stop" technique and the thoughts will resubmerge.

EXERCISE 49 "Stop" Technique

Directions: Use this exercise to help you overcome self-defeating thoughts.

1. List the thoughts that you use to put yourself down or that are self-defeating:
   a.
   b.
   c.
   d.
   e.
2. Take the first thought on your list. As soon as that thought forms in your mind, say loudly and clearly "Stop!" If the thought does not stop, say "Stop!" more loudly and firmly until the thought recedes.
3. Now say "Calm," and relax the muscles in your body for a moment.
4. When you can stop the thought, force yourself to have the thought, and then say "Stop!" again, loudly and clearly.
5. When the thought stops, say "Calm," and relax your muscles.
6. When you have mastered thought stoppage by verbal means, begin to *think* the word "stop." It may help to close your eyes and concentrate on the word "stop." When the thought stops, say "Calm," and relax your muscles.
7. Go on to the next thought on your list and repeat steps 2–7.

Occasionally, the "Stop!" technique will not work for especially recalcitrant thoughts. In this case, put a rubber band around one of your wrists and snap it and say "Stop!" when a self-defeating thought occurs.

Systematic Desensitization

Systematic Desensitization is a method you can use to reduce your reaction to upsetting situations. This procedure helps you develop a hierarchy of situations leading up to the upsetting event taking each situation and breaking it down into its component steps. For example, if you are extremely anxious about speaking up in a conference, you might construct the steps between waking up and thinking about the conference to the actual moment of speaking. The hierarchy might look something like this:

1. Waking up
2. Remember a conference is scheduled.
3. Driving to work and thinking about speaking up in the conference.
4. Arriving at work and seeing the conference schedule.
5. Noticing it is time for the conference.
6. Entering the room where the conference will be held.
7. Sitting down in the conference room.
8. The conference begins.
9. Getting ready to say something during the conference.
10. Speaking in the conference.

Go to Exercise 50 and complete it now.

EXERCISE 50 Systematic Desensitization

Directions: Look at the situations below and rank them from 1 (most distressing) to 14 (least distressing), then follow steps 2–4.

___ Telling others what I expect from them
___ Asking others what they expect from me
___ Saying no
___ Taking a compliment
___ Praising others
___ Admitting a mistake
___ Telling others about their mistakes or limitations
___ Asking for help
___ Standing up for my rights
___ Disagreeing with others
___ Expressing anger
___ Dealing with others' anger
___ Handling a put-down or teasing
___ Asking for a legitimate limit to my workload

EXERCISE 50 (*continued*)

Step 2: Choose the least distressing situation and construct 10 steps (see sample hierarchy above) from least fearful or anxiety-provoking (10) to most fearful or anxiety-provoking (1).

10.
9.
8.
7.
6.
5.
4.
3.
2.
1.

Step 3: Now think about being in the situation described in number 10. Visualize the situation in your mind. If you experience no anxiety or fear, think about the situation in number 9. If you begin to feel anxious or fearful, stop and practice deep-breathing and muscle relaxation (see pp. 000–000 for a sample relaxation script). Do not move to the next item in the hierarchy until you feel no anxiety when thinking about the event you are focusing on. Continue up the hierarchy until you feel no anxiety or fear when thinking about all the hierarchical steps you listed.

Step 4: Begin to try this process in real-life situations. Use the same procedure described in Step 3.

Affirmations

Affirmations are thoughts you have or words you say. How often have you said "That's the way things are," or "She'll never change," or "This won't work out"? Frequently, beliefs are just other people's opinions. If you were taught early in life that the world is a safe and joyous place, you probably believe that people are friendly, money comes easily, and love is all around. As a result, your life experiences mirror these beliefs, or at the very least you look for and pay attention to events that bear out your ideas.

You probably don't sit down and question your beliefs, but if you did you would begin to identify what motivates you and what your major perceptions of life are. If you listen to what you say for a week and write down the sentiments that you say more than three times, you will begin to understand your worldview. If anger, revenge, hurt, or worry rule your thoughts and words, that is what you will find. The way to have more control over your life is to change your words and thoughts.

Here are some positive thoughts to balance your negative thoughts that may be holding you back. Say or write one or more of the following thoughts at least 20 times a day. Write them on 3 x 5 cards and keep them in prominent places—your refrigerator, desk, dashboards.

- I love and approve of my life.
- I trust the processes of life.
- I am safe.
- My feelings are normal and acceptable.
- I am filled with love and understanding.

Guided Imagery

Guided imagery, or visualization, is another way to decrease your fear of anxiety about upcoming situations. In this procedure, you picture yourself acting assertively in a situation and then reward yourself for the fantasized act. It is recommended that you practice the imagery while you are totally relaxed and in a quiet, safe environment.

Self-Coaching

Self-Coaching is another procedure to use to decrease anxiety and fear. You may have found that when you get anxious, you get even more anxious when you realize you are tensing up. One way to handle this situation is to realize that signs of anxiety (such as sweaty palms and increased heart rate) are the same signs as for anticipation and excitement. Realizing this, you can coach yourself to relax by saying, "I'm excited about this situation, and that's good because it will help keep me alert and interested. I can control how excited I get. I will handle the situation one step at a time. I won't think about my fear. I'll concentrate on what I have to do. This will be over soon, and I can manage until then. It's not the worst thing that can happen. I'll concentrate on breathing deeply and easily."

Here are some other self-coaching statements to use:

- I can handle this.
- There's nothing to worry about.

- I will not allow this situation to upset me.
- I will take a deep breath and relax.
- I can take this step by step.
- I will take a deep breath and relax.

You may wish to write your own coaching statements. Carry them with you to read when you get into anxiety-provoking or fearful situations. Be sure to congratulate yourself after the situation is over and to remember that you *did* get through it.

Handling Backlash

Even if you learn all the assertive procedures well, you will have difficulty implementing them if you do not consider what effect your changed behavior will have on others. It is important to anticipate how others will react to your newfound assertiveness and to take action to deal with these reactions. With any change, others will resist and attempt by others to make you revert to the old familiar behavior or relationship. For example, coworkers or supervisors who have grown comfortable and obtained secondary rewards from protecting you or from watching you blow up and express their anger for them may feel betrayed or as if something is missing in your relationship with them.

Something *will* be missing—your dependency on them and theirs on you. Others may have an entirely distorted idea of what assertiveness is all about. To them, assertiveness may mean aggressiveness, and they may be uncomfortable once they find out you are learning about or practicing assertive skills. Others may dislike the short-term effects of having to adjust, but they may greatly appreciate your directness in the long run. Still others might surprise you by being delighted or pleased that you have taken the first step toward direct communication, because now they can feel freer to act on their goals. Often, others' appreciation or interest in assertiveness is camouflaged in confrontations or derision. So when you change, you can be fairly certain that your coworkers, family, or friends who knew you before will be surprised, bewildered, threatened, or delighted.

By not being threatened by others' comments and by educating them about assertiveness in a neutral, friendly way, you can ease change. You can also initiate talk about assertiveness. Tell coworkers and supervisors that you are learning to be more assertive and that the purpose is to enhance your skills. Once important people in your life have a better understanding of the skills you are striving for, they will be less fearful that you plan to change or outwit them. As with other teaching or learning processes, acceptance of information may require time and patience on your part.

Another technique to use is to enlist their help as partners in your practice. As an example, suppose your supervisor has just completed an evaluation interview with you and has said that you need to complete your work on time. At that point you may agree that you're concerned about this issue, that you are learning ways to do just that, and that you would appreciate help in role-play situations. If your supervisor agrees, you can set up time to practice role-playing in handling interruptions and in asking for help in setting priorities. You can tell your supervisor any rewarding messages you would like to hear, explain the rationale for using it, and ask that the message be said to you at specific times. In this way, you will not only develop a specific support for your assertive work, but you can teach your supervisor assertive skills indirectly. By taking the responsibility on yourself and presenting the project as something you are working on, you can decrease your supervisor's resistance. On the other hand, if you go around trying to convince others that they should learn to be more assertive, you are apt to increase their suspicions and resistance.

You may not feel comfortable enough to engage your supervisor yet. That is fine. You decide the situations you wish to be assertive in.

Besides letting the people around you know that you're working on assertive skills, it will be helpful (and often mandatory) to find at least one person who agrees to be your partner, who will read this book and participate with you in the practice exercises. That way you will both have the same knowledge base. That person can aid you in implementing skills in assertiveness by role playing problematic situations and planning strategy regarding how to approach a particular situation.

Yet another way to prepare for backlash is to think of remarks others might make and practice responding before you encounter them. Some model responses follow.

Model Response 1

Other: I don't mind that you're taking assertiveness classes, but don't try to change me.

You: I won't try to change you. I just want to be able to speak up and say what I want to say.

Model Response 2

Other: So, you're practicing being assertive. Are you learning how to arm wrestle?

You: Not at all, but I would like to talk with you about being a representative on the next committee that needs a member.

Model Response 3

Other: I don't like pushy people.

You: I'm not trying to be pushy. Assertiveness means setting goals, acting on them, and taking responsibility for my actions.

Model Response 4

Other: You really surprised me speaking up like that. I could never do that.

You: I've been working on saying what I think. Maybe we could do some role-playing together, then both of us could improve our skills in saying what we want.

Model Response 5

Other: You've changed. You don't ask for my opinion anymore.

You: I have changed and I miss our talks, too. Maybe we could have coffee together and I could tell you about the work I've been doing to reach my goals.

9
Gender Issues: Counteracting Patriarchy and Oppression

We don't see things as they are, we see things as we are.

—Anaïs Nin

Patriarchy and oppression can lead to a stress syndrome. Being female and a professional nurse complicates the picture further. Despite the negative environments that support patriarchy and oppression, there are positive actions you can take.

PATRIARCHY

Although women have made great strides in the workplace, if you're a woman you probably know that being a manager or administrator means floating in a sea of patriarchy. Women must battle for legitimacy in the workplace on a daily basis. It's an uphill fight. Men are often in power and they want to keep it. This is often true in the health care environment where most nurses are women and a majority of physicians and hospital administrators are men.

Nurses must endure the criticism most working women face, but they must also struggle with society's ambivalence about woman with power. Strong women are constant targets. Many people, both men and women, paint women who have power in unfeminine ways, as shrews who want to emasculate men. If you're an executive woman, you have probably been vilified by others who hope to control you by this maneuver.

A study of executive women (Gearing, 1994) found that no matter what business or occupation women are in, their worries, fears, and complaints fall into similar categories:

- Perception: They believe that because they are women, they have to give more 150% just to hold their own with male counterparts.
- Frustration and resentment: They are frustrated and resentful because they make one half to two thirds the income of their male peers.
- Restriction: They feel left out of the good-old-boy network.
- Anti-woman prejudice: Women who are not part of the power structure undermine women who are.
- Limitations: Executive women have few role models in the workplace.
- Humiliation: Harassment, sexual and otherwise, are constants.
- Unfavorable comparison: Women who work are often compared unfavorably to women who have chosen to remain at home.
- Exhaustion: Women who work often go home and take care of children and household responsibilities

MINIMIZING PATRIARCHY

Changing a patriarchy isn't easy. As the adage goes, the only thing you can change is yourself. That goes double for patriarchy. Seize the power you have. Go to Exercise 51 and see if you're suffering from patriarchy.

EXERCISE 51 Patriarchy

Directions: Check off the items below that apply to your environment. The more items you check, the more patriarchal your environment. Once you've identified the items, you'll be in position to decide which ones you'd like to change.

___ I must battle daily to achieve legitimacy.
___ A man is in power and refuses to give any to me.
___ People in my environment accuse me of being unfeminine, shrewish, emasculating, when I am assertive.
___ I have been vilified by others for being an outspoken woman.
___ I have to give 150% just to hold my own with male counterparts.
___ Although I do the same job as men in my job role, I get paid less than they do.
___ I am cut out by the good-old-boy network.
___ Women who are not part of the power structure undermine me.

(*continued*)

EXERCISE 51 (*continued*)

___ Powerful women are nonexistent or few and far between in my workplace.

___ I have to put up with harassment, sexual and otherwise, constantly.

___ I am compared unfavorably to women who have chosen to remain at home.

Now that I have identified the patriarchy of which I am a part, I have decided to work on changing the following item:

My goal to reduce this type of patriarchy is:

OPPRESSION

Do you feel oppressed? Does it seem as if another group or work system is holding you back or holding you down? Oppression can lead to low self-esteem, to anger and even violence against colleagues, and to passive-aggressive behavior. None of these reactions are assertive, but they are understandable.

Duchscher (2001) found that newly graduated nurses in acute-care settings felt oppressed, but they did not actively engage in addressing abusive behavior. That may be because oppression is a system problem, not an individual problem, although individuals may show symptoms of the syndrome. Exploitation often leads to symptoms of burnout. When you feel oppressed, you keep trying to achieve more and more in order to prove your worth. If you're a manager, you may lose your caring qualities and get lost in overseeing finances (Cullen, 1995).

When you're oppressed by another group, you may find yourself directing your anger at your colleagues because it isn't safe to direct it at the group that's oppressing you. As a result, you may be openly angry, negative, or sarcastic to your colleagues. Passive-aggressive behavior, an indirect expression of anger, occurs if you're oppressed and may show itself by undermining your peers or manager (Cullen, 1995). If you work in a setting where you're never allowed to show your best work or give your best effort, you are working in an oppressive environment. Complete Exercise 52 now and identify the cause and effect of oppression.

EXERCISE 52 Oppression

Directions: Identify the attributes of your environment that are oppressive. Decide on a goal to eliminate or at least reduce the oppression.

___ I am constantly being held down from achieving my potential.
___ Because I am oppressed, I don't think much of myself or my abilities.
___ Because I am oppressed, I take my anger out on my peers either directly or indirectly.
___ I try to achieve more and more in order to prove my worth.
___ When I feel oppressed, I find myself undermining my peers or supervisors.

The one oppressive behavior I'd like to change is:

STRATEGIES FOR REDUCING PATRIARCHY AND OPPRESSION

What is the antidote to patriarchy and oppression? Finding the best coping strategies and developing a blueprint for success is the answer. Coping strategies that have been used successfully by women and men in patriarchal and oppressive environments include forming strong friendships and social networks, learning to express your feelings, using an androgynous approach, centering yourself, exercising vigorously, avoiding self-blaming, nurturing and guarding your self-esteem, pursuing a strong commitment to your profession or business, using an assertive problem-solving style, and taking an action-oriented approach (Gearing, 1994).

Form Strong Friendships and Social Networks

Isolation is your enemy. Even though you may feel suspicious of others in your environment, you must force yourself to develop strong friendships and social networks. By investing in social networks, you will effectively insulate yourself from the negativity of patriarchy and oppression.

You will need at least several true friends who can form a mutual support system, be a resource for venting problems and finding solutions, and with whom you can relax and be honest. Even the best of friends can let you down once in a while. Be tolerant. Anticipate that there may be a disappointment or a let-down or two. Friendship is a gradual process and one that deserves nurturing.

If a friend disappoints you, analyze what happened and find a way to prevent it from happening again. Always make sure you are not in relationships that waste time and use you. Be sure your friendships include a point of connection and common ground so you can understand each other's situation.

The friendships must be honest and forthright. Social chitchat is a waste of your time. The feeling of being understood that comes from great friendships is invaluable and priceless. It validates your experience and breaks the sense of isolation that may be surrounding you. Friends can help you put your problems in perspective: Work is only 8 or so hours a day, the rest of your time is yours to do with what you want. Make sure you don't forget that. Learn French, start a garden, learn a new dance step, or read a classic on your time off. It will enrich your life and help you put patriarchy and oppression in perspective.

Talking with friends can help you see that your problems are similar to theirs. Talking things out can also help you begin to identify solutions because it helps you clarify what's in your mind.

Friendships can add balance to your life by allowing you time to let your hair down, relax, share fantasies, and reflections (Gearing, 1994). Friendships can also take the heat off your relationship with your partner or spouse. Expecting all things from one other person puts too much stress on a relationship.

Learn to Express Your Feelings

Whether you learn to express your feelings with friends or a therapist, find someone you trust with whom you can share them. The most successful women in Dr. Sylvia Gearing's study of executive women were the ones who were passionate and expressive. If you're in a situation where you believe it is not safe or helpful to express your feelings, it is still important to be aware of them. Avoid letting your feelings get trapped in your body. This can lead to pain and other chronic reactions you do not want or need. Instead, choose your venting situations and know when to pull back (Gearing, 1994). Refer to Exercise 53 for further assistance.

EXERCISE 53: Healthy Feeling Expression

Directions: Check off the situations in which you identify and express your feelings. If you're not engaging in any of these behaviors, write at least one specific goal for initiating a new behavior related to healthy feeling expression. Format and examples of this process include, By tomorrow, I will identify at least one person I can safely share my feelings with; and, By next Tuesday, I will develop a list of common feelings and carry it with me; or, By Friday I will take time to look at my list of feelings and reflect on when and if I felt any of those emotions.

___ I have given myself permission to acknowledge the emotions I feel.
___ I can identify the effect emotion has on my internal body processes. (stomach upset, headache, tense muscles, shallow breathing, dry mouth, cold hands, backache, etc.).
___ I have drawn up a list of common feelings from hope to hopelessness.
___ I carry a list of common feelings with me to remind me to pay attention to my internal processes.
___ Whenever something happens, I ask myself how I'm feeling about what just happened.
___ I take time each day to reflect on how events in my life are affecting me.
___ I have drawn up a list of people I feel safe sharing my emotions with that doesn't include my secretary, assistant, or boss.
___ I have experimented with sharing my feelings by picking an innocuous situation and sharing a positive feeling (joy, liking, pleasantness, etc.) with one person on my Safe to Share Feelings With list.
___ Now that I have found a friend I can safely share my feelings with, I am sharing my emotions and reactions to events.
___ I am having difficulty identifying my feelings and have made an appointment with a nurse psychotherapist, social worker, or psychologist to help me identify emotions.

My goal for identifying and/or expressing my feelings is:

Use An Androgynous Approach

If you work in a patriarchal environment, you may feel pressure to conform to the "male" style of processing information or communicating. By becoming more logical, analytical, or linear in your thinking, you close off another part of yourself that can be useful.

Doubting your impressions and feelings results in discarding these important bits of information about your environment. It is empowering to validate the emotional side of yourself, to accept that yes, you do have feelings and they are important in helping you hone your edge in a patriarchy. Keeping a sure hand on your empathy can polish your other skills and transform you into the ultimate practitioner or manager. Women who are the most successful embrace their feminine and masculine sides and integrate compassion and fire into their interactions, depending on which is appropriate.

Centering is a procedure that can help you integrate all sides of yourself into a whole person, with both "masculine" and "feminine" characteristics. Centering can help you achieve a base of stability. Exercise 54 provides information on how to center.

EXERCISE 54 Centering

Directions: Either ask someone to read the directions to you slowly, pausing for a minute after each ellipsis, or read the directions into an audiotape and follow them.

1. Sit in a comfortable chair with your feet flat on the floor and your hands resting quietly in your lap . . .
2. Close your eyes . . .
3. Check your body for tension spots . . .
4. On the next inhale, send a wave of relaxation . . . maybe as a color . . . to any of the tension spots you have identified . . .
5. On the next exhale, release any tension . . . perhaps as another color . . .
6. Continue inhaling and sending a wave of relaxation to tense areas . . . and exhaling and releasing tension until you feel relaxed and inwardly still . . .
7. Gradually, and without effort . . . allow your breathing to move to your center . . . about the level of your navel.
8. Picture all parts of you integrating into a whole person . . .
9. [Optional] Picture your body surrounded by a protective shield that allows positive energy in, but keeps negative energy out . . .. This shield can be conceived as a color or a light source.

Exercise Vigorously and Regularly

Regular and vigorous exercise is a strong antidote to stress, depression, and hopelessness. The most effective women in Gearing's study (1994) were more active and exercised at least several times a week. Although depression and apathy can make exercise seem like the last thing you want to do, push yourself and you'll find you come back from a session feeling invigorated and full of energy.

Defining yourself physically can empower you and raise your mood. You will stand more powerfully in the workplace when you are firm and energetic, adding a new kind of power to your repertoire.

The physicality that exercise provides, especially if you combine walking with free weights, can strengthen you, dispelling the of powerlessness many women feel about the violence toward women in this society. If you travel or work after dark, you are vulnerable to assault. Having your own physical perimeter defined and strengthened can increase your sense of potency, strength, effectiveness, and mastery. You will walk differently, hold your head higher, and be able to move quickly to avoid attack. As your body firms and moves with more agility, you send a powerful message to others that you are a formidable adversary. Complete Exercise 55 now.

EXERCISE 55 Using Exercise to Empower Me

Directions: Check off the items below according to where you are in your exercise regime. When you finish, examine your answers and write at least one exercise goal for yourself. Some examples are, I give myself permission to exercise and reap its benefits; I will begin exercising 3 times a week starting next week.

___ I have given myself permission to exercise and reap its benefits.
___ I exercise at least 3 times a week.
___ I have defined the perimeters of my physical space.
___ My body is becoming firmer and stronger.
___ After I exercise, I allow myself to feel an influx of energy and mood elevation.
___ I stand more powerfully on the ground.
___ My strengthened body now allows me to feel potent, effective, masterful, and strong.

My exercise goal is:

Avoid Self-Blaming

The most successful women in Gearing's study (1994) didn't blame themselves for the problems occurring around them. The less successful women resonated with the chaos and hostility around them. They bought into the fallacy that they were to blame for the problem. Besides being doubtful, it is also grandiose. Assuming that you might be the source of a system of anarchy is a distortion of reality. Instead of buying into these assumptions, use your time thinking about how to solve the problem, not wasting your time and energy berating yourself for having failed.

The successful women accepted responsibility when it was realistic and did not automatically assume they were to blame when a problem occurred. They sought solutions and didn't wallow in self-doubt or confusion. They didn't berate themselves, nor did they shoot from the hip, or force an immediate response from others. They controlled their impulse to answer immediately and didn't speak until they'd thought through their answers. By focusing on resolving the conflict, they got out of their own way and were successful. Behaviors that worked best included deliberateness, diplomacy, and well-considered action. Successful women were expressive in a self-controlled and shrewd manner. Complete Exercise 56 now to see where you rate on self-blame.

EXERCISE 56 Self-Blame or Responsible Action

Directions: Check off the items below that examine self-blaming behaviors and responsible action. After you identify responsible action, congratulate yourself. After you identify self-blaming behaviors, set a goal to help you toward responsible action.

Responsible actions:

___ I avoid blaming myself whenever a problem occurs.
___ When a problem occurs, I start thinking about how to solve it.
___ I accept responsibility when it's due and move on.
___ I know and use conflict-resolution skills.
___ I know how to be deliberate, consider all the facts, and be diplomatic.
___ I hold my tongue until I've thought about what I want to say.
___ When I do express myself, I do it in a self-controlled and shrewd way.

(continued)

EXERCISE 56 (*continued*)

Self-Blaming Behaviors:

___ If something goes wrong, I assume it's my fault.

___ When chaos and hostility break out, I have difficulty not feeling stressed.

___ I rush to fix things and believe I should be able to control everything around me.

___ When things go wrong, I expend a lot of energy telling myself I've failed again.

___ I wallow in problems and can't seem to find my way out.

___ When I'm upset, I shoot from the hip or try to force people to answer me.

___ I tend to act before I think.

Here are some examples of realistic goals for avoiding self-blaming:

• I will count to 10 before I shoot from the hip or try to force someone to answer.

• Instead of berating myself when something goes wrong, I will write down three ways I can handle the situation in the future.

Now it's your turn.
My goal for responsible action:

Nurture and Guard Your Self-Esteem

To be successful, you must learn to trust your own judgment and perception of reality. Doing this will nurture and guard your self-esteem. It will help you maintain a cohesive sense of yourself so you won't internalize the stress around you despite disruptions in your environment. When you trust your own judgment you can listen to other's opinions and not automatically buy into them. Your judgment is sound enough for you to make your own decisions.

No matter how healthy you are, you still may distort reality at times. It's only human. When you have nurtured and guarded your self-esteem, you are able to weigh what is said to you and interpret the motivation behind the words. Ask yourself, What does this person need, how does this person feel, and what is really happening in this situation?

While you're learning to interpret situations, be kind to yourself. Realize it will be trial and error for a while.

Be careful choosing your work team. Form a team that collaborates well. You deserve to surround yourself with the best people you can find. Make sure you select people based on sufficient data. Pay attention to and track situations, jotting down information as you gather it. Be especially aware of hidden agendas people have that could conflict with getting the work done. Pat yourself on the back when you accomplish something. Don't disregard your talents or accomplishments. You may be the only person available to nurture you so be sure you provide this needed reward. If you're less than pleased by your performance, remind yourself you put your best effect forward and that's the most important thing (Gearing, 1994). Many aspects of a work system are not under your control. Talk positively to yourself, censoring out any negative self-talk.

Pursue a Strong Commitment to Your Profession or Company

Gearing's study found that the most successful and healthiest women had an emotional investment in their profession or business. They had not lost that spark of interest and felt good about the work they were doing. Not everything worked out perfectly, but they cared about day-to-day operations, both successes and failures. These positive feelings about the workplace provided an important buffer against stress. Complete Exercise 57 now.

EXERCISE 57 My Commitment

Directions: Check off your reactions to each item, then select an appropriate goal.

____ I am emotionally involved in my work.
____ I feel good about what I'm doing at work.
____ I feel good about where I'm working.
____ I care about what's happening at work.
____ I feel I am part of whatever happens, both successes and failures.
____ I feel as if we're all working toward a common goal.

If you were unable to check all items, you may wish to discuss your career goals with your present employer or colleagues. It could simply be a matter of making others aware of your displeasure and planning a new role that could make the difference. Select at least one goal from the list below.

(continued)

EXERCISE 57 (*continued*)

1. I will take the following action to involve myself more deeply in my work:

2. I will take the following action to feel good about my work:

3. I will take the following action to feel good about where I'm working:

4. I will take the following action to ensure I care about what's happening at work:

5. I will take the following action to feel a part of whatever happens at work, both successes and failures:

6. I will take the following action to make sure we're all working toward a common goal at work.

You may have taken your time, been patient, and tried out all the steps you can think of to be happy in your work, and you still feel isolated and dissatisfied. Gather as much evidence as you can that there is no way to achieve your personal goals in the workplace you've chosen. If you conclude that you will never achieve your goals, it may be time to make a job change. Finding work in an unbiased workplace that supports your goals and dreams will be much healthier than remaining in an oppressive, patriarchal setting with no chance for promotion and little personal power.

Use an Assertive Problem-Solving Style

Less successful women in Gearing's study (1994) used an aggressive, confrontational style of problem solving. Many women chose a pushy approach when they were faced with an oppressive patriarchal work setting. Nevertheless, women were more successful when they avoided unnecessary confrontation and used diplomacy and negotiation instead. Gearing (1994) points out that in order to be an effective manager, you must manage the people around you or they will manage you.

Begin to monitor your tendency to be aggressive and confronting and to blurt out whatever occurs to you before thinking it through. Such a style may make you feel temporarily better because you've blown off steam, but later you may regret your display of uncontrolled emotion. Also, remember that the work setting is not meant to be completely open and all-trusting.

The most successful women in Gearing's study (1994) were versatile, adaptable, willing to change with speed and efficiency. They avoid proven formulas and are willing to step out of black-and-white thinking. They don't expect other employees to conform to their work styles. Instead, successful women modify their style of management to each employee's or each client's needs. With time crunches and scant resources, this may seem like a tall order, but it can occur. Put on your thinking cap and consider each problem a personal challenge to your creative ability rather than an infringement on your rules.

An important part of this style is keeping the larger picture in mind. Is it worth it to lose a skirmish in order to meet your long-term goals? Remember that being powerful does not mean being loud and confrontational. Many powerful people are quiet and thoughtful. They measure their words carefully and act when they are ready in a deliberate, swift, and effective manner. Try to emulate this style.

Ask for feedback regularly and use any remarks you receive to modify your performance when needed. Complete Exercise 58 now.

EXERCISE 58 Using Feedback

Directions: Check off the items that describe what other people have told you about yourself. If you're not sure how your colleagues and employees see you, consider giving them the list of the characteristics below and have them anonymously check the ones they think apply to you. Although it may be humbling, if a majority of your staff or colleagues give you the same feedback, come to grips with it and set goals to change your behavior.

___ pushy
___ aggressive
___ always blowing off steam
___ shares too many feelings
___ doesn't listen
___ out of control
___ unclear goals
___ black-and-white thinking
___ expects everybody to conform
___ impulsive
___ explosive

Based on the items I checked, I plan to take action on the following goals to bring my behavior in line with a consistently assertive approach:

Goal 1:

Goal 2:

Goal 3:

Goal 4:

Take an Action-Oriented Approach

To take an action-oriented approach, you must be clear about your goals, unapologetic about yourself, and able to embrace life fully (Gearing, 1994). If you feel paralyzed and overwhelmed by life, you will feel helpless, not life-embracing. If you are hurting and allow that hurt to consume you, there is no way to embrace life. If you allow problems in your life to affect your self-esteem, you won't be able to embrace life. When you feel good about yourself and act on your own behalf, you can live life to its fullest and be productive.

Even if you have suffered a lot of pain in your life, you can still learn how to enhance your self-esteem. If you are determined, you can shape and nourish yourself to be any way you want to be.

According to Gearing (1994), women don't get promotions because they don't get as many opportunities to prove themselves. Another reason could be that women don't always take the necessary risks because they're too busy to look up and see the bigger picture. Because women still carry a majority of the home and child responsibilities in our society, they must be uniquely organized to hire the right caretaker for their children so they have the freedom they need take action. To do this, mothers must be willing to give up any guilt they are carrying about not being home with their children.

One action that is necessary is for women as a group to advance the formalization of the "old-girl-network." The workplace can be a political game and women need mentors to show them the way.

Women often defeat themselves by not supporting each other. The trick is to support one another and simultaneously support men so there is no backlash that can threaten everyone's progress. Mentoring is another important aspect of bringing the old-girl-network into play. It includes helping other women understand how the mentor achieved her position and having frank discussions about the gender bias that exists in the workplace (Gearing, 1994). If you've been mentored, or even if you haven't but have learned a great deal in your career climb, actively think about grooming younger women for leadership.

REFERENCES

Cullen, A. (1995, November). Burnout: Why do we blame the nurse? *American Journal of Nursing, pp.* 23–27.

Duchscher, J. B. (2001). Out in the real world. Newly graduated nurses in acute-care speakout. *Journal of Nursing Administration, 31,* 426–438.

Gearing, S. (1994). *Female executive stress syndrome.* Ft. Worth, TX: The Summit Group.

10

Strategies for Career Enhancement

Don't worry and fret, faint-hearted, the chances have just begun, for the best jobs haven't been started, the best work hasn't been done.
—Berton Braley

To gain satisfaction in your work, it is vital for you to identify your assets, learning needs, and goals. Some indicators that you lack assertiveness in these areas are being passed over for promotions or leadership positions, performing work that should be done by others, and not being able to complete your work by the end of the day.

One reason you may be passed over for positions in leadership is that you have not thought your job goals through or considered what actions you need to take to move closer to that position. Or you may be a very competent practitioner, but others take credit for your actions and you never let important people know about your special skills. If it seems that you do all the thinking and work on the job yet no one recognizes it, you have a problem in assertiveness in this area. Another reason why you may not be sought out as a leader is that you are unable to mobilize your potential. You may procrastinate and never complete tasks on time. Supervisors or bosses often become frustrated with this kind of behavior and may wonder why you cannot achieve more. This pattern may be a carryover from school days when you waited until the last minute to complete an assignment and stayed up all night to complete it.

Another assertive difficulty in this area is constant complaining. If you constantly complain about work demands, the environment, or the way you are treated, but never think about what you can do to change the situation, you need skills in assertiveness. Yet another difficulty is being exploited. You may feel that you are over-worked and unrewarded. If this is the case, you probably have not learned to say no to unreasonable requests. As a result, you may experience bouts of crying and/or angry outbursts at work and annoyance and depression at home. The result may be an impulsive and sudden change of job.

Many of these problems may be due to not thinking through the role of a job. It is probably quite easy for you to see the economic importance of your job, but have you evaluated what you want to give to the job and what you want to achieve? It not, you probably will not gain what you want and may feel constantly dissatisfied with what you get. One factor that can interfere with setting assertive work goals is a learned conflict between being nurturing and goal-directed or problem solving. If you find yourself being pulled in two directions (wanting to be supportive and understanding, but also wanting to get on with the task and complete the work), you may be a victim of this unhelpful learning pattern. If so, you may need to become more aware of the conflict so you can find a constructive way to resolve it.

SETTING REASONABLE JOB GOALS

One of the first assertive steps to take in assessing job skills and goals is to examine which of the possible reality goals takes precedence for you. Some reality goals are earning a living, making as much money as possible, glory, status, prestige, reward for special skills, personal growth, and social contribution. Your reasons for choosing job goals are the same as for other assertive acts: You want to increase your self-respect and to move toward where you want to go in your life.

When you do not chart your professional goals and actively choose where you are going, you are choosing *not* to choose. If you want to be assertive, you have to develop goals. Job goals will give you a sense of purpose, which will motivate you to move toward meeting them. Once you achieve a goal, your self-esteem and self-respect will rise. You will begin to feel that you are moving through life purposefully rather than being propelled or resisting movement.

Setting long-term goals includes asking yourself the following:

- What kind of professional life do I want to live?
- What family, social, and other interests do I have that must be considered in goal planning?
- What dreams do I wish to achieve?

Moving toward a goal involves change. There is no getting around that. If you fear or resist change, it will be more difficult, but not impossible, to achieve your goals. If anxiety, fear, or resistance are part of your struggle to achieve your goals, look through the index and table of contents for specific sections that will help you manage your stress about change.

Remember that change has the potential for bringing you increased self-esteem and self-respect. It also means giving up old patterns of behavior or making a trade-off between the advantages and disadvantages that change brings. For example, if you decide to go back to school, you will have to give up some socializing, some old behavior patterns, and some earning power, at least temporarily. These are trade-offs. Every advantage carries a disadvantage. It is important to specify your goals and make decisions actively based on the advantages and disadvantages of each goal.

The other important element in planning your goals is in identifying your limitations. Your dream might be to open your own successful business or practice, but if you are fearful of striking out on your own or have no money or management skills, your chances of attaining that goal are minuscule. You have to be critical in looking at yourself as a person. You will limit yourself if you procrastinate and decide that a change is not worth the trade-off. Even if you procrastinate, you can still decide you want to change, and if you make a plan and work towards it, you will see results.

Some people are uncomfortable with the idea of planning long-term goals. They ask, How can I plan 10 years from now when I don't know what will happen next week? That's true, but if you don't plan, you can't be prepared. Granted, some events may intercede, but having a long-term goal can be reassuring during rocky times. Goals bring order to your life and help balance the insecurity of the unknown.

You may choose to stay at your current position and attempt to meet your job goals. In this case, you may decide to seek out and participate in additional educational experience to help you maintain skills and learn new ones. You may even decide to obtain an additional degree while continuing to work. Many degrees are now available on-line so you can obtain them without leaving your current position.

If you decide to leave your current position, search on-line for employment opportunities and read the information posted carefully, making sure they meet your requirements. At the same time, read classified ads in major newspapers and journals, and tell key people in your field that you are looking for a job and what your special qualifications and aspirations are. Learn the art of resumé writing and interviewing or create a job for yourself by starting your own practice or business or by convincing an agency that it needs your skills. Start by writing down everything you do in your current job. This will begin the process of identifying the skills you have mastered.

Whether you decide to stay in your current position or leave it, having short- and long-term goals can decrease work frustration. If your short-term goals are not working out, you can sometimes gain a sense of satisfaction by using that time to plan or work toward your long-term goals. For example, if your dream is to have your own practice or business, you can work toward that on your time off while still keeping your salaried position. This will allow you to have an income until your dream business takes hold and becomes profitable. The common-sense axiom about not putting all your eggs in one basket is applicable to work goals. The other positive thing about long-term goals is that you can change them. You have time. Use Exercise 59 to help you assess your job skills and goals.

EXERCISE 59 Assessing Job Skills and Goals

Directions: This exercise can help you begin to assess your job skills and to plan short- and long-term job goals based on your skills and needed expertise.

1. Special skills or talents I have are:

2. Tasks I most enjoy doing are:

3. Tasks I least enjoy doing are:

4. Expertise I need to obtain includes:

(continued)

EXERCISE 59 (*continued*)

5. One thing I want to accomplish in my work life is:

6. Dreams I have for myself include:

7. Learning experiences I need to plan to achieve my dreams are:

8. Skills or goals I plan to attain this year are:

9. Dreams I plan to make reality this year are:

10. To attain my dreams, I agree to make the following trade-offs:

11. Learning experiences I need to plan so I can attain my dreams for this year are:

12. Skills or goals I plan to attain within the next 5 to 10 years are:

13. Dreams I wish to make reality in the next 5 to 10 years are:

(*continued*)

EXERCISE 59 (*continued*)

14. Trade-offs I will make to achieve my dreams for the next 5 to 10 years are:

15. Learning experiences I need to plan so I can attain my 5- to 10-year goals are:

Once you have chosen your work goals, it is necessary to take an active approach toward getting the job you want. The more education and special skills you have, the more options you have to choose from.

You may choose to stay at your current position and attempt to meet your job goals. In addition, for your professional growth and as a way to assist you in attaining your goals, you will need to seek out educational experiences that can give you the skills you need. Although you may be able to find courses offered at convenient places and times, they may not further your goals. Begin to weigh the advantages of convenience against the disadvantages of not meeting your needs.

DELEGATING TASKS

If you're not assertive, you may not delegate tasks even when you have assistants to delegate to. You may also think you're the only person who can do the job right, so why delegate? Two good reasons are because you can't do everything without becoming stressed, resentful, and burned out; and if you don't teach your staff how to do your job, who will do it when you're promoted?

Often people fear they might lose power, control, prestige, or satisfaction if they delegate the work. If you feel this way, begin to question this counterproductive belief. Write down examples of objective evidence you have that this fear is unrealistic.

Successful Delegation

Successful delegation includes the following:

- a clear statement, preferably in writing, of just what the job entails
  end results expected
  suggestions you have for completing the task
  what authority or responsibility goes along with the task
  when you want a progress report
  a specific time you expect the task to be completed
  some idea of how the outcome will be evaluated
- clarification with supervisees of what is expected.
- establishment of controls and checkpoints.
- reiterating your expectations as needed.
- rewarding/praising supervisees' positive movement toward appropriate behavior.
- ongoing dialogue with supervisees about how they feel about the task(s) and how they evaluate their work.

Points to Keep in Mind When Delegating

- Write a sample script with the words you want to use when delegating. Role-play or rehearse with a trusted friend or audiotape recorder until you feel comfortable.
- Delegate using a tone of voice that says, This is important and I expect you to follow through.
- Check with the people you've given an assignment to, validate that there has been an agreement or understanding of the assignment by either having them read and sign a specific assignment sheet or by asking them to repeat back to you the assignment as they understand it.
- Verbalize the time or date you will be checking back to evaluate their performance.
- Check back with the person at the time agreed upon.
- When checking with supervisees, find out exactly what has and has not been accomplished to date.
- Work out a plan for supervisees to complete the assignment. If you take over and complete the task, you are not teaching the delegatee to be independent; you are teaching dependence.
- Provide praise and direction as needed.
- Be consistent in word and action; it is the hallmark of trust-building.
- Remember: Leadership includes teaching management skills to others so they can learn to be effective.

Ask yourself the following questions about your delegating style or the kind of delegating style you wished you had:

- How effective are my relationships with office and secretarial personnel and other people I supervise?
- What would I like to change about my relationships with any of these people?
- What is my action plan for changing these relationships and when will I begin to implement it?
- Do the people I supervise know when I expect them to interrupt me and when not?
- What is my action plan for letting my supervisees know when I expect them to interrupt me, and when will I implement it?
- Do supervisees know what decisions they can make on their own and what decisions to bring to me?
- What is my action plan for letting my supervisees know what decisions they can make on their own and what decisions to bring to me, and when will I implement it?
- Do I think supervisees will not give me feedback about problems they're having on delegated tasks?
- What is my action plan for making sure my supervisees give me feedback about problems they're having on delegated tasks, and when will I implement it?
- Do I fear I might lose power, control, prestige, or satisfaction by delegating some of the work to others?
- How can I make sure I don't lose power, control, prestige, or satisfaction when I delegate tasks?
- Do I feel that spending time planning how to delegate tasks doesn't fit with my action-oriented style?
- How can I save time and train my staff as well by delegating tasks?

ASKING FOR HELP

Do you operate under the false assumption that you should be able to do any and all work you are assigned? You may be assigned an unreasonable work load, emergencies can occur that necessitate assistance from other before you can complete your assignment, or you may find you are unable to complete your assigned tasks due to other reasons. If this occurs frequently, you may need help in setting priorities or delegating tasks to others. If it happens infrequently, you need to be able to ask for assistance without feeling guilty. If you never ask for assistance, you may be operating under some counterproductive beliefs including the following:

- If I ask for help, that means I'm not a good person.
- If I were a better person, I could do whatever is asked.
- I should be able to meet all demands placed on me.
- I should be able to handle all emergencies and unexpected situations and still complete my full workload.

If you are trying to do more than is humanly possible, you are probably feeling frustrated, angry, exploited, and unsatisfied. If so, the first thing to do is examine the counterproductive beliefs that prevent your asking for legitimate help. A model response for asking for help appears below.

Model Response

You: It's 1 o'clock now and I won't be able to complete my assignment without help. What help can I get? [points out problem and asks for help]

Boss: I don't have anyone to help you.

You: I've looked at the schedule (points to schedule) and Jane comes to work at two o'clock. I suggest she take over my report. [suggests solution])

Boss: She needs to get filled in on what's happening.

You: I'll give her a report and then give one again when the rest of the crew comes in. [compromises and suggests solution]

Note: Not all requests or subtle hints for help are legitimate. In the following situation, the real problem is setting priorities and planning time effectively so the task can be completed.

Model Response

You: I see you haven't completed your assignment.

Supervisee: No, and I won't have time. People keep asking me to do this and do that.

You: Are you saying you need help?

Supervisee: I need a smaller assignment.

You: Let's look at your assignment. [shows assignment sheet to supervisee] It looks to me like you have a fair amount of work.

Supervisee: Some of the other people have less work to do.

You: That's true, but the work they have takes more time and effort. [gives rationale for assignments] I might be able to give you some help to plan your work so you can finish on time. [states problem]

Supervisee: Everyone interrupts me.

You: So, saying no to interruptions is a problem. I can help you with that. I'd like to meet with you tomorrow to practice ways you can deal with interruptions. Eleven o'clock is a good time for me. (suggests solution)

Supervisee: Okay, but I don't know how talking to me will change them.

You: It won't, but I have some ideas about things you can do so you will be interrupted less often. We'll do some role-playing and you'll get more confidence saying no. Right now we need to decide how I can help you today so you can get your work completed.

See Exercise 60 for some situations to use in asking for help.

EXERCISE 60 Asking for Help

Directions: There will be times when your workload is unreasonable or when you have not allowed sufficient time to complete your assignment or specified goals. At these times, it is reasonable to ask for assistance. This exercise will help you clarify your goals when asking for help and work toward achieving them.

Model Situation: Asking for Help

You had three emergencies today that will make it impossible for you to complete your assignment. As soon as you realize you are falling behind, you approach your boss to ask for assistance.

You: _____

Boss: Don't bother me now, I'm busy.
You: _____

Boss: I guess I can give you a minute.
You: _____

Boss: Listen, I don't have anyone.
You: _____

1. List work situations that have occurred or that might occur in which you would think it reasonable to ask for assistance.

   a.

(continued)

EXERCISE 60 (*continued*)

   b.

   c.

2. List any counterproductive beliefs you may have about asking for help.

   a.

   b.

   c.

3. Dispel each belief, then go back and revise your list in number 1 if necessary.

4. Write an assertive statement for each work situation you listed in which you think it is reasonable to ask for help.

   a.

   b.

   c.

WHEN TO CONSIDER CHANGING YOUR WORK

Do you feel overwhelmed, underappreciated, or just worn out by the daily grind? Are you under relentless pressure and do you find yourself in a chronic state of alert? Does your work have a hold on you and your health? Do you have less and less free time? Are you developing stress symptoms?

Take Charge

It may be easier to blame the job, your boss or the system, or even blame yourself, but you will be more empowered if you put your energies toward improving your work. Instead of talking about how you're being mistreated, talk about how you're going to make things better. Set goals and deadlines for taking action to meet them.

Use Negotiating and Wellness Measures As a First Step

If your job is overwhelming you, it may be time to consider changing your work. That may or may not mean changing your job. It could mean negotiating with your boss to set priorities for which of the many tasks you've been assigned can realistically be completed. It might mean using stress management, exercise, and nutritional approaches to reduce stress. If these measures aren't successful, you will have to make some tough decisions. You may need to ask yourself whether your health or your job is more important. This may lead you down the path of looking for different work.

Learn to Be Joyful in Your Work

You have two choices if your work is not satisfying: Quit, or make it more satisfying. One way to make your work more satisfying is to fall in love with what you are already doing. Look at it from a different perspective. See that you are providing a service and identify the good in what you do. Once you have developed a spiritual center, each act of labor can be viewed for its contribution to the cosmic community. No work is a job in this sense, but a sacred act. If your work is useful and does no harm to anyone, it can be holy work and become a meditation.

Some affirmations that may help you turn stressful work into a meditation follow. (Affirmations are positive thoughts you give yourself to balance the negative thoughts and situations you may encounter. Write the affirmations on 3 x 5 cards and place them in places where you will read them at least 20 times a day, including refrigerator, car dashboard, bathroom mirror, desk, etc.).

- I am developing a spiritual center within me.
- My work is just a job.
- My work is holy work.
- I am falling in love with my work.
- My work contributes to the cosmic community.

Trust Yourself

The degree to which stress can disempower you and cause health problems depends on how you perceive outcomes. Does the idea of resigning create an anxious feeling in you, even though you know you're overwhelmed and overstressed and that your assignments are unrealistic? Here is an exercise you can use to question counterproductive beliefs that not completing the assignments will be disastrous.

What will happen if I don't complete this assignment on time?
My boss will be upset.
Then what will happen?
I could be fired.
Then what will happen?
I won't be able to pay my bills.
Then what will happen?
I'll lose my apartment or house.
Then what will happen?
I may have to go live with my family or friends.
Then what will happen?
I'll have to look for other work.
Then what will happen?
I'll look for something I really want to do.
Then what will happen?
I'll probably be happier and less stressed.

JOB INTERVIEWS

You've decided you can't stand your job another minute or you see a position advertised that will better your life. All you have to do is get through an interview.

Make sure your resumé has these characteristics (Cardillo, 2002); It should be 1–2 pages long and includes any information that shows you have prior work experience. For each previous job you've held, list accomplishments, most interesting experience, and most marketable skills. Even if you've got more than 20 years experience, include only the past 15 to 20 years in your resume

The job interview should be an interactive process in which you and the employer gather information about the fit between your job skills, the position, and the work environment. Many people have the attitude that they should be thankful if someone hires them, but it's up to you to decide whether your self-respect and attainment of job goals are more important than an increase in commuting time, a geographical relocation, or the effort needed to convince an employer that your services are needed. Talk with your family and negotiate shared responsibility for household and child-rearing tasks. Striking a satisfying balance between work and home is one of the issues assertiveness will help you face.

Perhaps you have some conflicting and counterproductive beliefs that even though you work 40 or more hours a week, you should also be totally responsible for a household. If this is the case, you may decide to join a consciousness-raising group for married couples or single parents to work out this issue. Whichever you choose to pursue, it is vital to remember that you are in control of your job planning.

If you decide to seek a new position or if you are a new graduate interviewing for your first job, you may wish to consider the following ideas:

1. Anticipate the questions employers may ask you and use a tape recorder to practice answering them. You may want to rehearse answers to some of the following questions until you hear yourself sounding assertive: How come you haven't worked for 2 years? Why did you leave your last job? Why should we hire you? What special skills do you have to offer us? If we gave you the job, what would be your priorities?

2. Be aware that there are some intrusive questions employers or personnel workers may ask you that have nothing to do with the job. These questions pose an opportunity to practice assertiveness, but they are legal issues as well. Some questions that you may choose not to answer based on issues of assertiveness and current legal grounds are all questions about mental health treatment or consultation, alcohol intake, and drug use (although you may be requested to take a urine test); "female-only" questions about pregnancy, menstruation, and female disorders; requests for a general blanket release of medical records; and questions about depression or other mental health indicators. Because different laws are applicable in different states, you may wish to check the legal status of these issues before taking an interview. Or you may wish to refuse to answer these types of questions because they present issues in assertiveness.

3. Write questions you want the employer to answer and use the tape recorder (or role-play with a peer) to identify assertive question-asking. Some questions you may wish to practice are, What tasks are included in this position? What responsibility and authority will I have? What decisions will I be expected to make myself? Who is directly responsible to me? What can I expect from you in terms of support for my decisions? What is the salary range? What are the fringe benefits? What possibilities are there for promotion? How will my work be evaluated? Who will I be evaluated by? What happened to my predecessor? (or, if there was no predecessor) How did this position happen to be created? What recourse do I have if I have a grievance?

4. If possible, be sure that the employer has had sufficient time to review your resumé. Merely going over a resumé is not an adequate job interview. It gives neither you nor the employer enough information to make a total evaluation.

5. Be assertive in the interview by dressing in appropriate and comfortable apparel, by going alone, picking the most comfortable seating space available, sitting tall and confident, maintaining eye contact with the interviewer, listening to the employer's questions and answering them concisely, and asking specific questions about the job. Never leave an interview without knowing the employer's time frame for deciding to hire you.

6. Present yourself in an assertive manner by speaking clearly and firmly, not putting yourself down, and not giggling or shrugging.

7. It possible, ask to spend some time in the environment in which you will be working. Talking with someone in the personnel or administrative office far removed from the workplace usually will not give you important information regarding who you will be working with, what the physical limitations of the work environment are, and the atmosphere of work.

If you are planning to create your own job, the interview will be more a matter of selling your skills to a prospective employer or defining your area of practice. In the former situation, you will need to spend more time identifying your special skills. Complete Exercise 61 now.

EXERCISE 61 Job Interview

Directions: Besides providing a potential job for you, job interviews can also provide useful practice in presenting yourself as a job applicant, in assessing the interviewer's expectations, and in asking important questions about job responsibilities, authority, and benefits. This exercise can be used prior to a job interview as a role-playing practice situation.

1. Write assertive responses to the following questions:
   a. Why did you leave your last job?

(continued)

EXERCISE 61 (*continued*)

Your response:

b. I see you're married. What if you have children? How will that affect your ability to perform your job?
Your response:

c. What does your husband [father] do?
Your response:

d. What makes you think you're qualified for this job?
Your response:

e. What is this gap in your resume?
Your response:

f. I notice you're overweight (smoke, skirt is too shirt, hair is too long, you have a tattoo).
Your response:

2. In preparation for taking a job interview, role-play one of the following situations with a partner. Directions for your partner appear below the role-play situations.

a. You have an advanced degree and are interviewing for a position.
b. You have 10 years' experience in your specialty and are applying for a job that will further your career.
c. You have just completed your baccalaureate and are interviewing for your first position.

Directions for the "interviewer": Be sure to ask why the other role-player is qualified for the position, to question or make negative comments about your partner's educational background, and to be quite difficult in general. Remember, you are giving your partner valuable experience. If you make the interview too easy, you will not be allowing your partner to practice dealing with some of the problems that may be encountered in real job interviews.

(*continued*)

EXERCISE 61 (*continued*)

3. Read the want ads and other advertisements for positions you are interested in. Pick a position and compile a list of questions and statements you would cover if you were actually taking the interview. Questions:

   a.

   b.

   c.

   d.

   e.

4. Choose one of the positions advertised and take an interview. Evaluate the results and write what you learned that you can apply in future interview situations.

PERFORMANCE REVIEW

You're responsible for your performance evaluation, which means you need to know the standards on which you're being judged. Ask for a copy of the evaluation tool and study it in advance of your review. If your evaluation is based on your job description, make sure you have a current copy. Know in advance how each evaluation item will be defined.

Before you head in for your evaluation, take stock of what you've accomplished since your last review. Sit down with a calendar and remember one or more significant ways you performed each month. A better idea is to keep a journal of your work accomplishments as you go, then all you have to do is refer to it while being evaluated.

Follow the steps below for a stellar performance review:

1. If you didn't meet your personal or agency goals, be prepared with a reason for why you didn't. Describe positive behaviors you exemplified instead, or tell why something else took precedence and why it did.

2. Mention every instance in which you exceeded employer goals. Present specific examples, not general statements. Whenever you can, work in ways you gave superior nursing care and saved your employer money at the same time.

3. always portray yourself as an active team player who made a difference in the nursing care of your unit. Mention colleagues who contributed to your success, but avoid making yourself sound like a passive follower who only performs well when coached or supervised by others.

4. If your evaluator brings up an error you committed or an area you were found lacking, ask for specific examples, then ask: "What do I have to do to change your perception of my performance?" Even better, come up with ways to change yourself and elicit validating from your evaluator that your evaluation would be enhanced had you acted that way or plan to act that way in the future.

5. When an error or lack is pointed out to you, acknowledge it and show how you learned from your mistake. Always thank your evaluator for any feedback, for example, "I appreciate your feedback."

6. If your evaluation is primarily negative and you don't agree, ask to write a written response to it and then provide specific examples of how you met employer expectations. Remember, silence indicates you agree. Stick to the point and always avoid blaming someone else (colleagues, supervisors, or the evaluator) for the evaluation.

7. Find someone outside of your workplace with whom to vent your feelings about your evaluation.

8. Use any comments from your evaluator that indicated lack or errors on your part. Set a personal goal for each comment so your evaluation improves the next time (Zurlinden, 2002).

PROMOTION

There are several ways to let others know about your special skills. Making your employer aware of your skills is the first step toward being considered for a promotion or raise. Make it easy for the employer by gathering data that show you should be promoted or rewarded. Keep records of procedures you have developed, leadership you have provided, research you have completed or contributed to, interventions or solutions you have developed or tried out, changes you have implemented, and any other actions you have taken to improve the organization's status.

Write a report of your work or a short position paper on an objective you have met. A combination of verbal and written documentation usually carries more weight than using one method only.

Find out what policies exist for raises or promotions. In many cases, employers have some options regarding hiring and promotion, although they may not always volunteer that information. If you can convince an employer that your work is valuable and needed, you will have a better chance of being rewarded by a promotion or raise.

Do your homework. Practice convincing arguments. Role-play or use audiotape or videotape replay to ensure an assertive presentation of yourself. As in other assertive actions, your request will not necessarily be granted just because you are assertive. Employers may not be assertive in return. They have a choice to be assertive, aggressive, or avoiding, just as you do. Your greatest rewards may come from feeling good about speaking up.

STARTING YOUR OWN BUSINESS OR PRACTICE

You may decide you can't provide the services or products you wish to in an agency setting. This may lead to an investigation of starting your own business or practice.

Taking on a new identity is confusing and trying, but it can lead to your becoming a more complex person with a greater understanding of your hopes, dreams, and goals. Part of taking on a new identity is accepting the instability in the world around you. Create your own stability in your life by exercising daily, eating right, getting enough sleep, and taking time to nourish your spirit and soul.

Use your support network. Let everyone know that you are thinking about starting your own business or practice and that in the meantime you are searching for a position that suits you. Give specifics about what you want. Enlist their help and ask for their ideas. Then listen, absorb, plan your strategy, and congratulate yourself on your enthusiasm and self-confidence. Ask current and former colleagues for ideas, too. Don't forget your mentors. Call them and let them know what's happening with you.

If you don't have a support group or mentors, create imaginary ones. Make a list of people you admire, then write a dialogue with them about your career and what steps they would use or suggest. Also, go to chat rooms on the Internet and business and professional associations in your community. Many chambers of commerce have regular networking meetings. Go there and talk to as many people as you can. Have a simple business card made up that gives your name and phone number or e-mail address and some of your skills and goals, and hand one out to each business person you talk to. If you don't have a card, be sure and collect their cards and ask if you can call them should you have questions later on. Follow up with each one who seems interested and supportive.

Repackage yourself. Take a pencil and paper and write down your areas of expertise. Be as specific as you can be. What do you do best? What do people tell you is your greatest strength? Use what you find out. Do you have teaching, creative, athletic, argumentative, friendship, intuitive, decision-making, leadership, teaching, mathematical or computer, observational, or calming and spiritual skills that you love to use? (refer to Exercise 59, for ideas). Can you sell your services or contract with companies to teach classes? Can you get testimonials and performance evaluations to back up your expertise? Talk to friends who work as consultants or trainers to find out the appropriate charge for your services.

If you opt to go it alone, you will have to struggle with the following issues: the laws and restrictions in your state, whether to rent or buy office space, financial concerns, liability insurance, legal counsel, accounting services, bank account procedures, partnership versus corporation, record-keeping procedures, needed consultation, fees and billing procedures, public relations and advertising, quality performance procedures, the development of a brochure and business cards to explain available services, secretarial services or answering service, what policies to establish, and what supplies and equipment are needed. Each of these issues can be anxiety-provoking and requires an assertive approach to result in a successful practice or business. You may never have questioned how much your expertise is worth per hour, how much your product is worth to potential buyers, how you will handle nonpayment situations, or how to deal with the anxiety about being out there, alone.

The following are some counterproductive beliefs you will need to dispel:

- It's too late to start over again.
- I'll never be able to get through interviews or selling myself.
- Who's going to hire me and want my skills?
- I shouldn't mention fee because it may turn potential off clients.
- I should be embarrassed to think my services or products have a price.
- I can't charge very much because no one will pay it.
- If a client doesn't pay on time, I shouldn't mention it.

These are assertiveness issues. Once you've dispelled your counterproductive beliefs, find a partner and role-play your responses to specific client and supplier responses until you feel comfortable dealing with each one.

CHANGING WORK HABITS

If you have difficulty establishing effective work habits, you may wish to use behavioral contracting to remedy that. Some common work habit problems include being late to work, not being able to concentrate on one task at a time, inability to complete written reports or records, or procrastination, you may choose to follow a seven-step procedure for changing work habits.

1. Identify the habit that must be changed. Behaviors must be pinpointed so that you can count or measure them. For example, behaviors that would not be countable are procrastinating, lack of concentration, or inability to complete reports. For the latter case, the countable behaviors are sitting at a desk in a quiet area, taking no phone calls, and allowing no interruptions. Once behaviors are specified, it's easier to set a course of action.

2. Count the pinpointed behaviors (baseline phase). This phase tells you where you are now and can be used as a comparison for determining progress. For example, how often each day do you sit at a desk in a quiet area every day for a week? How often do you refuse to take a phone call or stop an interruption every day for a week? These kinds of questions will provide a basis for counting types of behavior. Another aspect to consider is duration of the behavior. For example, how long did you sit at a desk or spend time refusing requests to answer the phone or to be interrupted?

3. Study the chain of behavior. Once baseline data are in hand, you can chart the chain of behavior that leads to your inability to complete a report or record. You may find the point at which your procrastination begins to gather momentum. For example, you may find you're able to concentrate until a friend calls with the latest gossip. Identify the events and people that play into your procrastination.

4. Make a contract of your intent to change. Be specific. For example, in the case of writing reports, a contract might be as follows:

I, _____ [your name], agree to spend 30 minutes every work day in a quiet area, sitting with the report data in front of me.

Your signature:

Date:

Although writing a contract makes it more official, you can also use a verbal contract. Tell your intention to a peer, someone who can monitor whether you fulfill your contract. Be sure to pick someone who is neutral about the contract, who will neither praise you for your intent nor scold you for it. Choose an intention you can accomplish in the near future, and aim for a series of successes. For example, gradually increase the time you expect to spend sitting at the
desk with the report.

5. Make it increasingly difficult to participate in the unwanted act. Make it difficult to procrastinate and easier to complete the desired act, in this case, complete the report. Shape your behavior in the desired path by rewarding yourself for completing the contract and by devising ways to entice yourself to complete the desired behavior.

6. Identify elements of your environment that tend to reinforce your unwanted behavior and remove them. In many instances, other people reinforce the undesired behavior. For example, other people may reinforce your procrastination by paying attention to it and commenting on it by saying, "Hey, what happened to your report?' or "You shouldn't be doing that, you should be doing your report." When you begin to procrastinate, others may ignore the change, thus withdrawing their reward (reinforcing it by paying attention to it), and making it less profitable for you to complete the report. For this reason, you must try to remove any situations that reinforce the unwanted behavior. Ask others to refrain from commenting on your behavior until you complete the report (desired behavior). If you cannot enlist their cooperation, you may be able to override their comments. One way to do this is to write yourself a firm message to remind yourself about your contract.

7. Select rewards. The last step is to establish the desired behavior. This step calls for selecting rewards to maintain the behavior. Rewards can be social (a pleasing interchange with friends), personal (buying yourself a favored object or food or treating yourself to a treasured experience), or usual (doing something you tend to do often so that you associate the new behavior with the older, familiar patterns). Be sure to reward yourself only after you have completed the desired behavior, and do it immediately. Keep records of your progress and post them prominently. Just having a concrete, visual sign of improvement will promote your continual practice of the desired behavior. As you begin to procrastinate less, plan to make it a little more difficult to obtain your reward. When you attain your initial contract with yourself to spend 30 minutes with the report data, increase the contract to 35 or 40 minutes, and add the stipulation that you will allow no interruptions.

REFERENCES

Cardillo, D. (2002). Resume writing. [On-line]. Available: www.nursingspectrum.com

Foster, D. G., & Marshall, M. (1994). *How can I get through to you?* New York: Hyperion.

Zurlinden, J. (2002). Preparing for a performance review. *Nursing Spectrum, 12,* 6–7.

11

What Nurse Leaders Can Do

We could never learn to be brave and patient, if there were only joy in the world.

—Helen Keller

There is a lot more to being a nurse leader than knowing how to apply theory. If you've been in administration or management for a while, you've already learned that. Congratulations! If you've learned the lesson, but are still a little bewildered about what to do, or if you're new to the management mantle, read on.

USE EMOTIONAL INTELLIGENCE

Emotional intelligence guru Daniel Goleman outlined ways to manage with the heart and still get the job done based on *Emotional Intelligence at Work* (Weisinger, 1998). Let's take a look at two ways to handle the same situation. Which way do you think will win your staff's kudos and which will result in undermining and backsliding?

Situation: Your assistant has badly handled a client and you're livid. There goes your credibility and his. You storm into the room where he is sitting with five other employees and say one of the following:

Response #1:

Why in the world did you do that? You must have half a brain in that head of yours. What you did was just plain stupid! One more trick like that and you're fired!

Response #2:

Good morning. Can I speak to you alone? [Then, after you're in a private area] I noticed you spoke with Mr. Justin about the work schedule for today. Let's take a look at it together and see if we can't come up with an alternate plan.

Bring a sense of optimism to your management messages by focusing on the circumstances and how they can change, rather than on the negative characteristics of the person (Bobulski, 2002). This will take some of the heat and emotion out of situations and provide a learning experience, not a trial by fire, for your staff.

That's for the short term, the everyday, specific situations. What can you do to unite your work team in the long run? You have to connect with them. Here are some tips (Bennis, 1989):

1. Be there when it counts. Let your staff know where you are and make sure you're in the trenches when trouble explodes.

2. Be supportive during a crisis. Don't focus on what the situation means to you, but on what it means to your team.

3. Don't just talk about caring. Show you care. Even if you're angry, take a moment (or longer if needed) to compose yourself before you speak. Make sure you own your anger and focus on the problem, not on your feelings.

4. Avoid surprises. Prepare your staff for changes by helping them talk about how the change can affect them (don't just tell them how it will), and by encouraging them to actively participate in the change (not simply to adjust to it). This takes time and adjustment to change takes time, that is if you don't want a rebellion—either active or passive—but it's well worth the effort.

USE RESEARCH RESULTS TO SUPPORT YOUR ACTIONS

From software engineers (Perlow, 1998) to teachers (Koustelios, 2001), and even in a diverse sample of employees drawn from a variety of organizations (Eisenberger, Cummings, Armel, & Lynch, 1997), research has demonstrated that leadership can positively or negatively affect performance and job satisfaction. Being encouraged to communicate and being rewarded for doing so has been correlated with greater satisfaction and greater perceived organizational influence (Avtgis, 2000). Perlow (1998) found workers harried by competing demands, frequent interruptions, and shifting deadlines. Koustelios (2001) found the teachers were dissatisfied with their jobs when they lost their personal identity or suffered emotional exhaustion. Eisenberg and colleagues (1997) showed that perceived organizational support was highly correlated with job satisfaction for employees in a wide variety of organizations.

Taormina and Law (2000) asked 154 nurses in five Hong Kong hospitals to complete the Maslach Burnout Inventory (MBI), and Organizational Socialization Inventory (OSI), and three measures of personal stress management. Nurses who had high job training, organizational understanding, coworker support, and future prospects had the least burnout. Nurses who knew personal-stress-management measures were less likely to feel depersonalized and they were able to accomplish their goals more easily than nurses who didn't have these skills. Without strong interpersonal skills and coworker support, there was apt to be a decreased sense of personal accomplishment. Based on these findings, check off at least 4 goals from those that follow and set a date to accomplish them.

___**Encourage workers to communicate their ideas and reward them for doing so.**
Date to accomplish:

Dates to monitor program effectiveness:

___**Ensure there is a weekly support group to provide coworker support to decrease emotional exhaustion and enhance personal identity.**
Date to accomplish:

Dates to monitor program effectiveness:

___**Hire a consultant to teach employees personal stress management skills.**
Date to implement:

Dates to monitor program effectiveness and plan additional workshops if needed:

___**Provide all employees with information about future prospects and changes.**
Date to accomplish:

Dates to monitor program effectiveness:

___**Survey employees to find out their training needs and then plan classes to achieve them.**
Date to accomplish:

Dates to monitor program effectiveness:

Nurses identified high workload, low influence over work assignment, limited avenues for skills development, and diminishing support from supervisors as sources of considerable tension resulting in deterioration of work conditions and decreased job satisfaction (Severinsson & Kamaker, 1999). Lewis (1999) found that implementing an oncology staff bereavement program reduced staff burnout. A recent survey conducted by a physician (Rosenstein, 2002) of 1,200 nurses, doctors and hospital executives in 84 facilities found that more than 30% knew nurses who had left hospital nursing because of doctors' behavior. Intimidation, possible retaliation, and confidentiality concerns were cited among reasons nurses did not report physicians' disruptive behavior. Financial cutbacks, scheduling and mandatory overtime were also perceived as factors in staff shortages.

A study of social workers, community nurses, and community psychiatric nurses (Parry-Jones et al., 1998) found that an increased workload and administrative duties combined with reduced opportunities for client contact were their main sources of stress. Being able to control or shape those factors lay at the heart of stress and job satisfaction.

High levels of stress and the challenges of working with critically ill children and their families can threaten job satisfaction and result in job turnover of nurses in pediatric critical care units. Bratt, Broome, Kelber, and Lostocco (2000) surveyed 1973 staff nurses in 65 institutions in the U.S. and Canada. They found that management strategies are needed that empower staff to provide quality care and that diminish the stress caused by nurse-family interactions.

Clear and open communication is a crucial skill for nurse managers to support and role model. If you can't confront verbally abusive doctors, how do you think your staff will learn? With fewer young people choosing nursing as a career, it becomes mandatory to keep those already in the profession from leaving due to physician abuse. Other factors identified by Rosenstein's research (2002), including financial cutbacks, scheduling issues and mandatory overtime must also be tackled if you wish to maintain a high quality staff. Although all nurses receive some education in communication skills, only psychiatric and mental health nurses focus on this aspect in their work. Managers who wish to decrease staff stress and empower their staff will have to learn communication skills if they do not possess them. Even if you think you possess good communication skills, it would be wise to attend an assertiveness workshop with or without your staff. By demonstrating your willingness to learn new assertive skills, you will more likely convince your staff that it is not only safe but useful to attend an assertiveness workshop.

Not only nurses benefit from communication inclusion. Teachers (Koustelios, 2001), software engineers (Perlow, 1998), and workers in a multitude of organizations (Eisenberger, et al., 1997) benefit from inclusion and organizational support. Based on the research presented, check off at least four goals from the list that follows and include a date when you will implement them.

___**Implement a plan so employees have more influence over their work assignments.**
Date to implement:

Dates to monitor program effectiveness:

___**Devise a plan to ensure ongoing monitoring of supervisors so that they provide verbal and visible support for employees they supervise.**
Date to implement:

Dates to monitor program effectiveness:

___**Implement a plan to increase employee/client contact.**
Date to implement:

Dates to monitor program effectiveness:

___**Hire mental health nurse consultant to teach employees and clients interventions to reduce stress.**
Date to implement:

Dates to monitor program effectiveness:

___**Ensure that all employees attend an assertiveness training class or a 2-day assertiveness workshop.**
Date to implement:

Dates to monitor program effectiveness and plan follow-up consultations.

As organizational pressures mount, an increasing concern is how managers will meet both staff and organizational needs without burning out themselves. Leaders must show that their staff's best interests are their number one concern, they must be physically available and genuine (Fletcher, 2001). Use Exercise 62 to problem solve regarding how you can meet both employee and organizational needs without burning yourself out.

EXERCISE 62 Meeting Employee and Organizational Needs

Directions: Fill out all three columns. Make sure that you consider the burnout aspects for each behavior you suggest.

Employee needs	Organizational needs	How I will ensure both are met without burning out

You may need more information to solve the problems of your employees. A problem-solving format may help you gather the information you need. Figure 11.1 provides the questions to ask to begin this problem-solving process.

According to Phelps and Austin (1997), specific behaviors indicate whether an organization encourages assertiveness. Check off the encouraging signs that you will ensure are instituted in your organization and a date for their implementing related actions.

___ Start an **employee suggestion box** that is regularly read and implemented.

Date to implement:

Dates to monitor program effectiveness:

___ **Open up communication** so it flows up, down, and across all organizational levels, by starting a newsletter that shares information from all levels, including anticipated organizational changes, achievements and rewards.

Date to implement:

Dates to monitor program effectiveness:

FIGURE 11.1 Problem-solving format.

---

1. Definition of the problem
a. What is the nature of the problem as defined by the employee. ("Tell me what the problem is," and "What is the problem as you see it?" "Correct me if I'm wrong, but what I hear you saying is_____.")
b. How severe is the problem? ("What effect is the problem having on you?" "How is the problem making it difficult for you to do your work?" "How often does this problem occur?" "Let me see if I have understood what you said. _____.")
c. When does the problem occur? ("How long has this problem been going on?" "When does the problem usually come up?")

2. Determinants of the problem
a. What intensifies the problem? ("What makes the problem worse?" "What else is going on when the problem occurs?")
b. What decreases the problem? ("What is going on when the problem decreases?" "What have you tried to do that reduces the problem?")
c. What is the source of the problem? ("What do you think is causing the problem?" "What evidence or facts do you have to support your ideas?")
d. What precedes the problem? ("What brings the problem on?" "What sorts of things are going on when the problem surfaces?")
e. How are others handling the problem? ("What do your colleagues do when the problem occurs?" "What do your colleagues do to decrease the problem?" "What do your colleagues do to increase the problem?")
f. What effect is the problem having on your self-esteem and motivation? ("What feelings are you having about the effects of the problem?" "How is this problem affecting your motivation?" "In what ways are you being stressed by this problem?" "On the one hand, I hear you saying _____and on the other hand, I hear you saying _____. I wonder how these two things go together.")

3. Possible solutions
a. What are some suggested changes. ("What do you think should be done to improve the situation?" "Looking back, how could you have reacted differently to the problem?" "What is the best way to decide what to do?" "What would be a good back-up decision?" "What could you or I do to improve the chances of our being successful?")
b. Suggested further inquiry. ("What can I do to help you with this problem?" "What other information do you need to help solve this problem?" "What support do you need to help solve this problem?" "Let us consider how we might find out together." "We've covered a lot of ground. Is there anything I've said that was confusing or troubling?")

___ Begin an **Assertiveness Rewards** program that recognizes and rewards independent action and speaking up in constructive ways.
Date to implement:

Dates to monitor program effectiveness:

___ **Place more emphasis on performance than on status** by rewarding excellent performers with financial, educational, and other (depending on a survey of employees) rewards.
Date to implement:

Dates to monitor program effectiveness:

___ **Develop an open door policy** for employees that includes no fear of retribution for voicing complaints.
Date to implement:

Dates to monitor program effectiveness:

___ **Invite nonsupervisory employees to sit on decision-making committees.**
Date to implement:

Dates to monitor program effectiveness:

___ **Initiate regular sessions to ask for all employees' opinions** on work-related decisions, issues, products, services, and disagreements.
Date to implement:

Dates to monitor program effectiveness:

One study of 1,741 nurses (Bourbonnais, Comeau, & Vezina, 1999) and another of supervisory and nonsupervisory employees in a large Canadian teaching hospital (Brown et al., 1999) found that social support can mediate the stressful components of job demand and lack of control in the worksite.

Managers' leadership is crucial to critical care nurses' deciding to stay in a position. Communicating clearly with staff, allowing them to be autonomous, and supporting group cohesion decreased job stress and increased job satisfaction. Managers with leadership styles that seek out and value contributions from staff, promote a climate in which information is shared, promote decision making at the staff nurse level, and influence coordination of work to maintain stability were associated with retention of staff and decreased job stress (Boyle, Bott, Hansen, Woods, & Taunton, 1999).

Another study found that meeting training needs, protecting time for discussion, and improving two-way communication helped alleviate stress in nurses (Cooper, 1999). Fallowfield and Jenkins (1999) found that insufficient training in communication and management skills for oncologists and specialist cancer nurses was a major factor contributing to stress, lack of job satisfaction, and emotional burnout.

Klein's study (2000) found that nurses were stressed by the death of their patients and by witnessing suffering, but the highest level of stress was not related to patient care at all. Organizational problems such as interpersonal conflicts with coworkers, inadequate resources, and communicating with physicians were reported as the most crucial. The researcher suggested that nurses undergo skills training in conflict resolution and assertiveness to address their organizational difficulties.

A study of 10,700 employees found that counseling may be the method of choice for employees who have strong stress reactions despite low job stressors, show signs of family problems, request counseling, or have a need for psychiatric treatment (Kosugi & Otsuka, 2001).

REDUCE STAFF BURNOUT AND RETAIN EMPLOYEES

If you're a nurse manager or leader, there are many actions you can take to reduce burnout and retain employees. Many of these actions will not change the fact that staff is insufficient. Prior to helping heal others, you must first heal yourself. Give yourself permission to learn skills that will enable you to empower your staff. Take communication and stress-management courses until you feel empowered. Once you have evoked all the potential deep within you, begin to reap the benefits of your role modeling-ability by teaching your staff what you have learned.

Sharpen Your Communication Skills

Take a course in communication skills, conflict resolution, and assertiveness. Learn how to really listen to your employees. Listen to the words and the messages between the lines. Learn how to use empathic communication so you can support the thoughts and feelings of your staff, empowering them so they will want to do their jobs to their utmost ability.

Empower Your Employees with Needed Workshops

Provide assertiveness, communication, conflict resolution, stress management, and management workshops for employees. Staff will feel empowered if they know they can handle their own and others' stress, if they can communicate clearly and get the expected response, and if they know how to delegate tasks and use their time effectively. Make sure the workshops you choose offer actual simulated situations for your staff. Research has shown that the more practice situations are similar to real work situations, the greater transfer there will be to the work setting. When you make this type of learning experience available, your staff will see you as an excellent role model and manager and will be more apt to stay in their positions and be productive workers.

Set Up Support Groups

No matter how long the hours or how demanding the job, if employees feel support from you or their colleagues, they will work hard and long and feel empowered. At least one a week have a brown-bag-lunch support group session for workers. Allow no more than 12 workers per group. Tell them the purpose is not to complain or blame, but to provide support for one another. Make sure they've already had workshops in communication, assertiveness, stress management, and conflict management skills. Ask them to rotate each week, randomly picking one person to be the focus of their attention that week. Then ask them to spend the hour making suggestions to that person about how to handle whatever issues they raise. This will empower the person being focused on because they will receive total attention and also gather useful strategies, and it will empower staff because they will experience their power by helping a colleague.

Meet Staff Training Needs

Ask your staff what they want or need to learn to be effective in their jobs and then make sure you provide it either by bringing in a consultant or paying for on-line or in-school class work. This will not only provide information for you about their training needs but will empower them by increasing their ability to problem solve, be autonomous, and make decisions about what will affect them.

Be Physically Available and Genuine

Negotiate for an administrative assistant and train that person to do your paperwork, freeing you to be available to your staff. Spend time observing, talking with and asking for staff input. Train yourself to hold the opinion that your staff is competent and able to function competently. Being physically available without being able to provide support will be less likely to empower your staff to more efficient action so be sure to avail yourself of workshops and consultation that empowers you.

Teach Employees to Coordinate Their Work

Be sure to teach your employees coordination skills. If you need assistance learning how to do this, hire a consultant you feel comfortable with and role-play coordination situations until you feel empowered to help your staff coordinate their work. It will be well worth the effort to head off mix-ups that can stress everyone and waste valuable time.

Increase Employee Opportunities for Client Contact

Most, if not all, of your staff gains great satisfaction from client contact. If they are satisfied and feel competent, they will be efficient in doing the rest of their work. Teach them how to prioritize tasks and delegate nonclient duties. (If necessary, hire a consultant to teach you how to prioritize tasks, delegate nonclient duties, and teach your staff to do the same.)

Survey Employees About Their Job Stress

You may think your staff is handling their work assignments, but if you don't know how stressed they are, you may be overlooking a chance to head off dangerous eruptions of backbiting and even violence. At the least, you may be reducing health payments for staff whose stress has led to physical symptoms that increase sick days and decrease worker efficiency. You may wish to hire a psychiatric mental-health nurse practitioner to conduct a job stress survey. Employees who test high for job stress and low on coping strategies and social support could be referred for counseling or workshops teaching these skills.

Congratulate Yourself on a Job Well Done

Bosses may be the last people to receive compliments and emotional rewards. Your salary may be high (or not), but you may feel unappreciated by, and distanced from, your employees. No matter how hard you've worked to open communication channels, there will always be a distance between workers and employers. You hire, fire, and discipline them. You can't confide in them and although they may turn to you for help, you can't turn to them for personal reasons.

Because of this you must build in rewards and compliments for your own work well done. Institute a Treat Myself Today award when you've accomplished one of the goals you've identified. Treat yourself to a massage, a favorite movie, time in a special retreat or to some other activity that makes you feel renewed and inspired.

Be sure to seek out and spend time with supportive colleagues who are also in administrative positions. Ask for their help and consultation and even for a shoulder to cry on when needed. Write affirmations on cards and place them in strategic places so you will feel complimented. Some suggestions are *I did a good job and I appreciate me. I'm getting closer and closer to my work goals.*

REFERENCES

Affinito, M. G. (1999). *When to forgive.* Oakland, CA: New Harbinger.

Avtgis, T. A. (2000). Unwillingness to communicate and satisfaction in organizational relationships. *Psychological Reports. 87*(1), 82–84.

Bennis, W. (1989). *Becoming a leader.* Reading, MA: Addison.

Bobulski, E. D. (2002). A message for managers: Care teach, connect. *Nursing Spectrum, 12*(3FL), 9.

Bourbonnais, R., Comeau, M., & Vezina, M. (1999). Job strain and evaluation of mental health among nurses. *Journal of Occupational Health Psychology, 4*(2), 95–107.

Boyle, D. K., Bott, M. J., Hansen, H. E., Woods, C. Q, & Taunton, R. L. (1999). Managers' leadership and critical care nurses' intent to stay. *American Journal of Critical Care, 8,* 361–371.

Bratt, M. M., Broome, M., Kelber, S., & Lostocco, L. (2000). Influence of stress and nursing leadership on job satisfaction of pediatric intensive care unit nurses. *American Journal of Critical Care, 9,* 307–317.

Brown, J. A., Woodward, C. A., Shannon, H. S., Cunningham, C. E., Lendrum, B., McIntosh, J., & Rosenbloom, D. (1999). Determinants of job stress and job satisfaction among supervisory and non-supervisory employees in a large Canadian teaching hospital. *HealthCare Management Forum, 12*(1), 27–33.

Cooper, J. (1999). Managing workplace stress in outpatient nursing. *Professional Nurse, 14,* 540–543.

Eisenberger, R., Cummings, J., Armeli, S., & Lynch, P. (1997). Perceived organizational support, discretionary treatment, and job satisfaction. *Journal of Applied Psychology, 82,* 812–820.

Fallowfield, L., & Jenkins, V. (1999). Effective communication skills are the key to good cancer care. *European Journal of Cancer 35,* 1592–1597.

Fletcher, C. E. (2001). Hospital RNs' job satisfactions and dissatisfactions. *Journal of Nursing Administration, 31,* 324–331.

Goleman, D. (1994). *Emotional Intelligence.* New York: Bantam Books.

Hintikka, J., Koskela, T., Kontula, O., Loskela, K., & Viinamaki, H. (2000). Men, women and friends— are there differences in relation to mental well-being? *Quality of Life Resources, 9,* 841–845.

Klein, J. A. *Sources of nursing stress.* [On-line]. Available http://www.nursingnetwork.com/stress1.htm. Accessed ll/24/00.

Kosugi, S., & Otsuka, Y. (2001). Psychological counseling as a management of stress in the work place. *Sangyo Eiseigaku Zasshi, 43*(3), 55–62.

Koustelios, A. (2001). Organizational factors as predictors of teachers' burnout. *Psychological Reports, 88*(3 Pt. 1), 627–634.

Lewis, A. E. (1999). Reducing burnout: development of an oncology staff bereavement program. *Oncology Nursing Forum, 26,* 1065–1069.

McKay, M., Rogers, P. D., McKay, J. (1989). *When anger hurts, quieting the storm within.* Oakland, CA: New Harbinger.

Parry-Jones, B., Grant, G., McGrath, M., Caldock, K., Ramcharan, P., & Robinson, C. A. (1998). Stress and job satisfaction among social workers, community nurses and community psychiatric nurses: Implications for the care management model. *Health, Social Care and Community* 6(4): 271–285.

Perlow, L. A. (1998). Finding time, stopping the frenzy. *Business Health, 16*(8), 31–35.

Phelps, S., Austin, N. (1997). *The Assertive Women.* San Luis Obispo, CA: Impact Publishers.

Rosenstein, A. H. (2002). Nurse-physician relationships: Impact on nurse satisfaction and retention. *American Journal of Nursing, 102*(6), 26–34.

Severinsson, E. I., & Kamaker, D. (1999). Clinical nursing supervision in the workplace—effects on moral stress and job satisfaction. *Journal of Nursing Management, 7*(2), 81–90.

Taormina, R. J., Law, C. M. (2000). Approaches to preventing burnout: The effects of personal stress management and organizational socialization. *Journal of Nursing Management, 8*(2), 89–99.

Weisinger, H. (1998). *Emotional intelligence at work.* San Francisco: Jossey-Bass.

Let Me Know About Your Empowerment

I'd like to hear from you about your empowerment stories: what has helped you feel empowered and what obstacles you've overcome. Contact me at cccwellness@earthlink.net and visit my Web site at http://home.earthlink.net/~cccwellness for wellness tips and news about available and upcoming books, workshops, and consultation availability. Also send me information about other topics to include in future versions of this book.

Above all, be empowered! You deserve it.

Index

S *Springer Publishing Company*

Integrating Complementary Health Procedures into Practice

Carolyn Chambers Clark, EdD, RN, ARNP, HNC, FAAN

This is a practical guide to integrating comple- mentary/alternative therapies into a traditional health care practice. It can be used by physicians, nurses, mental health professionals, physical therapists -- anyone who wants to augment or enhance their services or simply understand what their patients may be doing on their own to help themselves. The first half provides rationale and strategies for making a blend of traditional and nontradi- tional practices work – such as overcoming

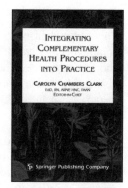

patient or colleague resistance, research corroborating alterna- tive therapies, insurance considerations, and marketing. The second half outlines actual therapies that can be used, chosen by the author from personal experience as those most likely to make a successful complement to traditional practice.

Partial Contents:
Part I. General Principles
- The Practitioner -Client Relationship
- Over coming Resistance to Complementary Procedures
- Evaluating Results
- Marketing a Complementary Practice

Part II. How to Integrate Selected Complementary Therapies
A. Nutrition, Herbs, and Essential Oils
B. Healing Systems
C. Mind/Body Approaches
D. Therapeutic Activities

2000   364pp   0-8261-1288-9   hard

536 Broadway, NY, NY 10012
Order on-line: www .springerpub.com • Order Toll-Free: 877-687-7476

Springer Publishing Company

Encyclopedia of Complementary Health Practice

Carolyn Chambers Clark, EdD, RN, ARNP, FAAN, Editor in Chief;
Rena J. Gordon, PhD, Contributing Editor
Barbara Harris, RN, LMT and **Carl O. Helvie,** RN, DrPH
Advisory Contributing Editors

This comprehensive resource of key terms and concepts in complementary health care addresses practices, conditions, and research-based treatments. With over 300 entries by distinguished contributors, coverage includes such alternative therapies as naturopathy, homeopathy, chiropractic, nutrition, and massage.

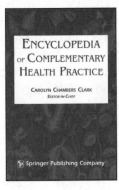

One section is devoted to pertinent issues in complementary health practice including economics, legal ramifications, education, and historical perspectives. Other valuable features are the extensive cross references and a directory of practitioners and institutes relevant to complementary health practice.

Partial Contents:
* A Theory for Complementary Health Practitioners
* The Role of Science in Complementary Health Care
* Complementary Health Practice: A New Paradigm
* The Economics of Complementary Health Practices
* Complementary Health Centers and Networks
* Complementary Health Practitioner Locations
* Effects of Complementary Health Practices on Medical Education
* The Education of Homeopaths
* Education and Research Conducted at CAMPS
* Legal Rules Affecting Complementary Health Practice: Malpractice and Vicarious Liability
* National Center for Complementary and Alternative Medicine
* Wellness Promotion: Historical Aspects
* Self-Care in American History

1999   664pp   0-8261-1239-0   soft • 1999   664pp   0-8261-1237-4   hard

536 Broadway, New York, NY 10012 • Telephone: 212-431-4370
Fax: 212-941-7842 • Order Toll-Free: 877-687-7476 • Order On-line: www.springerpub.com